Dr. Lazare's

THE PATIENT'S GUIDE TO BIOMIMETIC DENTISTRY AND SMILE DESIGN

This book is the *ultimate* guide to everything you would like to know, and everything you should know, about your dental health…

With topics that include:

- ➢ Biomimetic Dentistry
- ➢ Smile Design and Smile Makeovers
- ➢ Porcelain Veneers and other Cosmetic Procedures
- ➢ Teeth Whitening
- ➢ Dental restorations including veneers, bonding, Lumineers, crowns, bridges, inlays, onlays, and tooth-colored fillings
- ➢ Invisalign and Orthodontics
- ➢ Dental Implants and Oral Surgery
- ➢ Root canal treatment and how to avoid it
- ➢ Gum disease (causes and treatments)
- ➢ Preventative care and X-rays
- ➢ Alternative dental therapies
- ➢ Diet and nutrition for dental health
- ➢ How to keep teeth for a lifetime
- ➢ Dental emergencies – what to do
- ➢ Minimizing pain, fear and anxiety
- ➢ Children's dental care
- ➢ Geriatric dental care (elder care)
- ➢ Oral cancer prevention
- ➢ Medical conditions and oral health
- ➢ TMJ pain, tooth sensitivity, cracked and broken teeth, grinding, clenching, swellings, bleeding gums, cavities, bad breath, dental care during pregnancy, and much more…

The *ultimate* guide to everything you would like to know, and everything you should know about your dental health

Dr. Lazare's

THE **PATIENT'S** GUIDE TO BIOMIMETIC DENTISTRY
AND
SMILE DESIGN

Marc Lazare, D.D.S., M.A.G.D, F.A.B.D.

President of the Academy of Biomimetic Dentistry
Master in the Academy of General Dentistry

Order this book online at www.trafford.com
or email orders@trafford.com

Most Trafford titles are also available at major online book retailers.

Print information available on the last page.

ISBN: 978-1-4907-9869-1 (sc)
ISBN: 978-1-4907-9871-4 (hc)
ISBN: 978-1-4907-9870-7 (e)

Library of Congress Control Number: 2019920191

Trafford rev. 03/09/2020

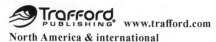

www.trafford.com
North America & international
toll-free: 1 888 232 4444 (USA & Canada)
fax: 812 355 4082

Dedications and Acknowledgements

This book is dedicated to my family, friends and patients...

Throughout my career I have been devoted to the pursuit of excellence, personal transformation and sharing of knowledge while exploring the world and living life to its fullest. Every person comes into your life for a reason. Some are a constant like my parents who I dedicate everything to, and my sister, Lauren, who has always been there for me, and others may be transient or lasting...like a specific teacher, lecturer, or friend whose words, suggestions, connections and examples can open your mind to the possibilities and help set you on a certain path. Then there are my children, Hunter and Sydney, who recharge my batteries, renew my love for life and give me purpose. I have others in my life too whose love, kindness and inspiration refills my cup everyday, allowing me to pour that love, kindness and inspiration into the cups of those around me. After all, you can only share what it is that you have. I am also very grateful to my late friend, Alex, who first introduced me to Biomimetic Dentistry in the early stages of this revolutionary movement and the mentors that have taught and inspired me. My life's goals are very similar to the tenets and principles of Biomimetic Dentistry...I try my best to stay vital and maintain all important connections, building layer upon layer on a strong and healthy foundation, doing everything possible to minimize stresses, creating beauty wherever it is lacking and getting bonded and then staying bonded to all that supports me.

Dr. Lazare's
THE PATIENT'S GUIDE TO BIOMIMETIC DENTISTRY AND SMILE DESIGN

TABLE OF CONTENTS

Dr. Lazare's
THE PATIENT'S GUIDE TO BIOMIMETIC DENTISTRY AND SMILE DESIGN

PREFACE:

Fun Fact...

A *smile* is our most powerful expression. It can turn any negative moment into a positive one in the blink of an eye.

The Facts

"It is important to know the tooth, the whole tooth and nothing but the tooth"

The world of dentistry has changed, and there is a great deal of confusion, conflicting opinions, and misinformation out there in the media. Fear of dentistry and lack of understanding about modern dental procedures, such as Biomimetic Dentistry, have resulted in many people failing to take advantage of the dental care necessary to help them keep their teeth for a lifetime.

With the onset of dozens of beauty and makeover television shows, and the attention that is given to those who have undergone these procedures, the average person no longer wants an average smile. The terms veneers, porcelain crowns, bridges and implants have entered into the common vernacular. People want to be more informed and more esthetically conscious. Every person is a dental patient. Everyone has a vested interest in learning their options and understanding what the latest technology has to offer them.

There are many questions people have about dental care. There are terms that they have heard mentioned but aren't quite sure what they are. They have heard about advances in dental technology and various treatments but don't know who to ask about them. Their dentist is often too busy to present all the different choices one has, and doesn't have the time to explain in detail what needs to be done. People have a fear of the unknown and a fear of dentistry is common. We all are concerned with doing what is best for us while trying to keep costs down. There are many aspects of basic dental care we do not understand. The idea of when to see a dentist, and if I go will I have pain, are just some of the universal concerns. Here, in one book, are the answers we need.

This book includes:

> ➢ Biomimetic Dentistry – a revolutionary form of dentistry
> ➢ Smile Design and Smile Makeovers
> ➢ Porcelain Veneers and other Cosmetic Procedures
> ➢ Teeth Whitening
> ➢ Dental restorations including veneers, bonding, Lumineers, crowns, bridges, inlays, onlays, and tooth-colored fillings
> ➢ Invisalign and Orthodontics
> ➢ Dental Implants and Oral Surgery
> ➢ Root canal treatment and how to avoid it
> ➢ Gum disease (causes and treatments)
> ➢ Preventative care and X-rays
> ➢ Alternative dental therapies
> ➢ Diet and nutrition for dental health
> ➢ How to keep teeth for a lifetime
> ➢ Top 10 ways to minimize dental costs
> ➢ Dental emergencies – what to do
> ➢ Minimizing pain, fear and anxiety
> ➢ Children's dental care – and teeth eruption charts
> ➢ Geriatric dental care (elder care)
> ➢ Oral cancer prevention

- ➢ Medical conditions and oral health
- ➢ TMJ pain, tooth sensitivity, cracked and broken teeth, grinding, clenching, swellings, bleeding gums, cavities, bad breath, dental care during pregnancy, and much more...

This book was written by **Dr. Marc Lazare**, the **President** of the **Academy of Biomimetic Dentistry**, **Master** of the **Academy of General Dentistry**, **Founder** of the **Lazare Institute for Biomimetics and Smile Design**, author of *Dr. Lazare's - The Patient's Guide to Dentistry*, and the creator of the popular *Dental Expert* and *Pediatric Dental Expert* apps for the iPhone and iPad. Dr. Lazare has gathered information from the top dental experts in their fields to answer the most frequently asked dental questions in all categories of dental care. *Dr. Lazare's - The Patient's Guide to Biomimetic Dentistry and Smile Design* is the *ultimate guide* to everything you would like to know, and everything you should know, about all aspects of cutting edge Biomimetic, Esthetic and General Dentistry. Dr. Lazare coined the phrase "Biomimetic Smile Makeover" in an article he published of the same name.

Dr. Marc Lazare is an internationally renowned lecturer, dental columnist, featured author in peer reviewed dental journals, teacher, consultant, inventor of two of the top instruments used in cosmetic dentistry, and President of Cosmetic Innovations, Inc. He is well regarded by his peers, recognized as an authority on Biomimetic and Cosmetic Dentistry and also known by many as 'Dentist to the Stars.'

1

BIOMIMETIC DENTISTRY

Fun Fact...

The tooth is the only part of the
human body that can't heal itself.

Mimicking Nature's Beauty,
Strength and Durability

"Get Bonded, Stay Bonded"

There has been a paradigm shift in the way dentistry is being
practiced. Those dentists at the top of their game and on the cutting
edge of new technology and techniques are now able to save their
patients' teeth and conserve their good tooth structure so much
more than before through a dental discipline we call Biomimetic
Dentistry. Biomimetic dentistry is tooth-conserving dentistry.
Literally translated 'Bio-mimetic' means to mimic life. We study
nature's properties so that we can better duplicate it. Biomimetic
dentistry treats weak, fractured and decayed teeth in a way that
keeps them strong and seals them from the invasion of bacteria.
It reduces the need for cutting teeth down for crowns and helps to
prevent root canal treatments whenever possible. In essence, it is
utilizing the latest in dental materials and technology to preserve
what we have, for as long as possible. In terms of materials,
techniques and skills Biomimetic dentistry can take aesthetic
dentistry to a whole different level of dental practice. Biomimetic

dentistry is not only about creating the strongest restoration, but rather creating a restoration that is highly compatible with the structural, functional and biological properties of underlying dental tissues. This revolutionary form of dentistry works by reproducing and emulating the original performance, characteristics and aesthetics of the natural tooth. It does take a different skill set, some new materials and protocols, a bit more patience and a certain amount understanding of the science behind the techniques.

Dentists need to shift the context of their thought process and rethink what is possible. They need to stop thinking about mechanically retaining restorations and start better understanding adhesion. No one should condemn a tooth that still tests vital. Just because a tooth had a root canal or has crack lines does not mean it needs a crown. To reach this new level of dentistry and clinical excellence we need to look way beyond the core techniques taught in dental school. Each patient has to be treated as an individual, and dentists must enlist the science and techniques of Biomimetic dentistry, and recognize that dentistry is the art of improvisation. With Biomimetic dentistry, we don't just fill teeth…we restore them. The most successful dentistry is comprised of procedures that are the least invasive. This is the philosophy and primary emphasis behind the principles of Biomimetic dentistry that we are proud to practice. For example, if a tooth is structurally compromised, we reinforce the remaining tooth structure with a polyethylene fibered mesh to disperse the forces imposed on the tooth when chewing… the same way a wire mesh is placed within a plaster wall to absorb the forces it may sustain. In Biomimetic dentistry we layer the esthetic, biocompatible bonding materials in a way that minimizes the stresses between the restoration and the tooth structure. This helps to prevent developing cracks that could lead to fracture, and protects the margins of the restorations from breaking down in order to seal out bacteria. The materials that we use mimic the elasticity and strength of enamel and dentin, and are layered to enhance the bond strength of the material to the tooth, minimize the stresses that cause a restoration to break down, and blend in the natural shades and characteristic of the original tooth color to make a final restoration that is difficult to find, even when blown up in high definition on a big screen.

The published article, "The Biomimetic Smile Makeover,", demonstrated just how one could conserve and strengthen tooth structure while transforming a smile. Rejuvenating one's smile has the power to inspire self-confidence and rebuild one's image. Invasive procedures and unnecessary reduction of tooth structure can eventually weaken the teeth and result in stresses and cracks, contributing to bacterial infections and fractures, and the subsequent need for root canals, extractions, implants and bridges. By adhering to the principles and fundamentals of Biomimetic dentistry, we can achieve uncompromised esthetic results and give our patients beautiful, healthy, and youthful smiles. This will help enable them to find new love, land that new job, give them that extra edge in business and networking, and live happier and healthier lifestyles.

Question: My dentist doesn't do Biomimetic dentistry, what should I do?

Answer: Once you are educated to understand the principles of Biomimetic dentistry it will be very hard to allow yourself to be treated the way you were before. Your mind will be opened and you will be armed with the knowledge that certain procedures, such as root canals, posts, crowns and extractions may be too invasive and aggressive for your needs, and often times your teeth can be saved using minimally invasive and more conservative techniques. As patients become more educated about their options, this will drive them to have the necessary conversations with their dental provider and hopefully pave the way for their dentists to look into taking Biomimetic continuing education courses and then incorporate them into their practices. You may also visit www.aobmd.org to search for a *Certified* Biomimetic dentist near you.

Question: How do I know if my dentist is a *Certified* Biomimetic dentist or just saying they are doing Biomimetic dental techniques but really just doing their regular traditional dentistry?

Answer: A Biomimetic dentist needs to be *certified* by the **Academy of Biomimetic Dentistry** as a "Biomimetic Dentist" in order to perform these procedures to the proper standards of care.

The kind of dental procedures that save tooth structure, prevent sensitivity, protect the vitality of the nerve, and stop the tooth-death cycle. In order to become certified, a dentist must have completed a certain number of continuing education courses in Biomimetic dentistry, passed their written exam and must have attended at least one of the academy's annual meetings. They must also remain a member in good standing, and pledge to ensure that the philosophy, theory and standard application of Biomimetic dentistry stays pure and aligned with the published peer-reviewed scientific literature and to apply its application to the best of their ability on each and every patient.

Question: Why wouldn't a dentist want to practice Biomimetic dentistry?

Answer: The protocols are technique-sensitive and more time-consuming and require a certain amount of continuing education, training and patience on the part of the dentist. Perhaps the dentist may be older and set in their ways or not fully understand the benefits at learning Biomimetic dentistry at this stage in their career. Dentists may also choose their traditional, more invasive and more aggressive dentistry because they can make more money by doing a root canal, post, core, crown and perhaps a crown lengthening periodontal procedure, knowing that the tooth is compromised and that the restoration may fail sooner than later. Once the tooth becomes compromised, and all that unnecessary dental work fails, they can then charge for the extraction, bone grafting, implant, abutment and crown. Conversely, Biomimetic restorations, techniques and protocols can, money, time and tooth structure and avoid unnecessary dental work.

Question: How are Biomimetic reconstructions different than regular tooth-colored bonded fillings and why might the prices be different?

Answer: While both Biomimetic reconstructions and regular tooth-colored bonded fillings rely on resin materials and adhesive technology, the protocols for Biomimetic dentistry are more technique-sensitive (requiring a more advanced understanding of adhesion) and use only the gold standard of bonding agents (according to unbiased published peer reviewed studies) and use materials that mimic the type of tooth structure being replaced. For example, Biomimetic dentistry will use materials that mimic the modulus of elasticity of dentin for dentin replacement, and materials that mimic the hardness of enamel for enamel replacement. Additionally, these stress-reducing Biomimetic protocols include utilizing polyethylene fibers to help scaffold the weakened, cracked and thinner walls to act as a structural framework that distributes the forces throughout the tooth/restoration complex. This is done in the same way a plaster wall is reinforced with a wire mesh inside so that when it gets hit, it doesn't break in that spot, but rather the forces get shared throughout to help maintain its integrity. In Biomimetic dentistry, the dentist is taught to build up the composite resin restoration layer by layer using small increments to avoid shrinkage and gap formation, which could contribute to bacterial leakage and sensitivity. Many dentists who do traditional dentistry just bulk fill the holes and use one material for replacing both dentin and enamel, even though the biologic properties are so different.

In dentistry, just as in many other service industries, time is money. These Biomimetic reconstructions take longer to perform and utilize better and more expensive materials to ensure the longest lasting bond and most comfortable and durable restorations. While you might be paying more for a biomimetic restoration than a traditional dental filling, you will most likely be saving many times more over time by avoiding the root canals, posts, crowns, extractions and implants that are inevitable with invasive dentistry.

Question: Do most insurance companies cover these Biomimetic dental procedures?

Answer: At this point in time most insurance companies do not recognize Biomimetic dental procedure codes…but hopefully that will soon change. Most dentists who are on the committee that decides which codes are reimbursable are either not well-versed in Biomimetic dentistry or are too old to have had the chance to practice utilizing these materials and protocols. Nothing worthwhile ever comes easy, and we all know the political red tape that goes on in Washington. It makes no sense that at this point in time Insurance companies would rather pay 50% or more of a root canal and a crown than pay less for a restoration that can prevent the need for root canals and crowns. Patients need to know that they would actually save more money (and tooth structure) paying for a Biomimetic restoration fully out-of-pocket than doing the unnecessary invasive dental procures that the insurance companies recognize and cover. However, there are codes that can be submitted to still get a decent amount of the cost of biomimetic procedures covered. Your dentist should know the best way to utilize your benefits.

Question: Are Biomimetic dental restorations biocompatible with the body?

Answer: Yes, Biomimetic dental restorations are biocompatible and mimic the biology of the natural tooth. Holistic and alternative minded patients can rest at ease knowing that in Biomimetic dentistry no metals are used (no amalgam restorations, pins, posts, etc.). This is the most natural, bio-emulating and conservative form of dentistry practiced today. Whether your Biomimetic dentist utilizes direct stress-reduced bonded restorations or indirect bonded restorations such as dental onlays, you can be assured that they are working hard to try to mimic the natural properties of your original tooth structure.

Question: Which types of invasive and costly procedures can Biomimetic dentistry save me from?

Answer: Biomimetic dentistry can save you from root canal procedures, (assuming the nerve is still vital), the cutting down of perfectly good tooth structure for crown and bridgework, the placement of posts within the canals of a tooth, (since these only

6

contribute to the fracturing of teeth), periodontal crown lengthening procedures, (since often times the deep margins can be elevated with certain bonded materials), and the unnecessary condemning of teeth for extraction, bone grafting and implants, since there is nothing better than your own tooth.

Question: Biomimetic dentistry talks about stopping the Tooth-Death Cycle...What is the Tooth-Death Cycle?

Answer: The excessive and often unnecessary removal of good, sound healthy tooth structure by traditional dental practices is what starts the tooth's ultimate demise; known as the "tooth-death cycle." While at one point in time placing a large silver-mercury amalgam filling was considered conservative, it is now recognized as one of the worst things you can do to a tooth in terms of undermining its structural integrity. Even tooth-colored fillings, when prepared in the same manner as the silver fillings, can sever the tooth's inner connections and undermine the tooth's supportive structures. Traditional dentistry relies on mechanical retention, where Biomimetic dentistry relies on the science of dental adhesion. In order to get mechanical retention, a dentist would need to drill down to a certain depth and remove and undercut the good sound tooth structure in order to physically retain certain non-biomimetic restorations. The reason why teeth with silver fillings crack and fracture is because they are undercutting good tooth structure and every time you chew or grind your teeth you are taking that metal wedge of a filling and placing an outward force on the thin walls of tooth structure, which will eventually cause them to crack and fracture. Additionally, silver amalgam fillings hold none of the tooth's dentin or enamel properties and do nothing to help restore the tooth's natural biomechanics, strength and durability. This is why biomimetic restorations and techniques should be the only way to reconstruct and restore one's tooth, since the materials used in Biomimetic dentistry mimic the natural characteristics of the tooth structure it is replacing.

The "tooth-death cycle" is as follows: A cavity is discovered and even if it is small, a lot of good, sound tooth structure is removed and undercut in order to receive traditional dental treatments such as a silver mercury (amalgam) filling. This significantly weakens the tooth. The stresses and grinding and chewing forces on this newly compromised tooth will, over time, contribute to crack formation and may cause a portion of the tooth to fracture. The tooth may now become very sensitive and the traditional dentist would initiate root canal therapy, (which removes the nerve within the tooth and makes the tooth more brittle), and then cut down even more perfectly good tooth structure all around in order to place a crown on the tooth. Often time when there is not enough tooth structure to work with or just simply because it is the cookie-cutter technique they teach in most dental schools, the traditional dentist would stick a large metal or ceramic post in that hollowed out root canal area that the crown now goes around. The result of this is an extremely rigid restoration that functions in no way like the natural tooth. Over time the chewing forces cause the root to fracture from the movement of the hard post within the center of the tooth, causing the fractured tooth to now be extracted, and grafted in preparation for a dental implant.

This entire "tooth-death cycle" could have been avoided if Biomimetic dentistry was utilized instead of traditional dentistry. In biomimetic dentistry the good tooth structure would have been preserved, and the materials used to restore the tooth would be completely biocompatible. The materials used to replace dentin would have the same modulus of elasticity as dentin and the materials used to replace enamel would have the same hardness as enamel. Other biomimetic materials and techniques are utilized to help restore the severed connections.

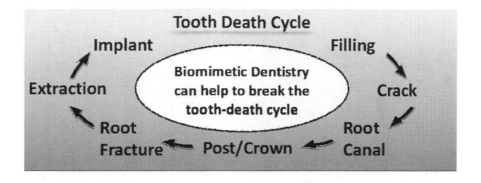

Question: What is Air Abrasion and what are its benefits?

Answer: The Biomimetic dental community is committed to practicing minimally invasive dental procedures. Our goal is to keep the pulp (the tooth's nerve) vital and preserve as much good tooth structure as possible. One of the more common techniques to do this is called Air Abrasion. Air Abrasion is a drill-free technique that can remove small areas of decay and stain to clean the surfaces of teeth. It works by blowing a strong mixture of air and tiny particles (usually aluminum oxide or a baking soda mixture) onto the tooth with powerful pressure while the tooth is isolated and the particles are rinsed and suctioned away.

Some of the benefits of Air Abrasion include no discomfort, vibration, heat or scary sounds while cleaning away small areas of decay. It may also reduce the need for anesthesia if the cavity is shallow, and there is no risk of chipping or fracturing any tooth structure. It also works very well on children and those with dental anxieties. Another great advantage is that tooth-colored composite material adheres very well to tooth surfaces that has been prepared and cleaned with Air Abrasion, helping to ensure longer lasting restorations.

2

SMILE DESIGN

Fun Fact...

The largest and most complex smile ever built was a giant smile created by the architect Alison Brooks in 2016 at the London Design Festival made from cross-laminated tulipwood and measuring 35 meters wide.

Creating structural harmony and optimum esthetics

"Design is where science and art break even"

Smile Design is not only about creating balance and harmony within a smile, but also has much to do with creating the illusion of perfection in asymmetric frames through utilizing various dental materials, designs and techniques. Smile design principles such as determining where the placement of the tooth's edges should be, the development of pleasing width/height ratios and the development of the esthetic contours of the tooth's gum line, should all be utilized to achieve the desired goals. In smile design even the smallest detail should have a meaning or a purpose. A mouth with narrow arches can be made to appear broadened by building out the ceramic or porcelain materials as we move towards the back of the mouth.

This decreases the dark empty space that once highlighted that narrow arch form. Teeth themselves can be made to seem larger or smaller, wider or narrower just by reshaping them to reflect the light differently. Modifying line angles can change the zone of reflection. A flatter surface will reflect more light to create a wider appearance, while tapering the edges will reflect less light causing the tooth to appear narrower. Incorporating surface texture and natural translucency can help absorb or reflect light to make the tooth look more polychromatic and natural. The chewing edges of teeth should also be given texture and character to make it appear that the patient has chewed with them before. For older patients, you can add some craze lines in these teeth to make them appear more natural. This is part of the artistry that goes into the design of a smile. Additionally, one can create a softer, more youthful and more feminine appearance just by reshaping certain corners of the teeth and by modifying their heights (i.e. making the side front teeth just a touch shorter than the two front ones). Rotating teeth can also add some natural qualities and give the patient back some of the character of their old smile that they felt defined them in a good way.

Question: How can one be assured that their expectations can be met with the design of a new smile makeover?

Answer: It is very important to have realistic expectations about what can be achieved with a new smile makeover. If steps are not taken for the patient to fully understand the process, they are not informed of any possible limitations nor able to visualize the end result, then the patients may sometimes find themselves in a place where they are disappointed with their new smile, despite all efforts to correct it. Even if the smile is objectively beautiful to others, it can still be considered a failure if expectations are not met. The person receiving the makeover needs to feel that their new smile matches their personality and who they are in order for the process to be considered a success. One very important step is to create a mock-up of the potential enhanced smile that the dentist can use to demonstrate what that future smile could look like. A putty template can be created from that mock-up in order to allow the patient to "try on" their potential new smile with a temporary tooth-colored material. This will help patients envision the possibilities and have realistic expectations about what can be accomplished.

Question: How does a cosmetic dentist handle asymmetry and customize and personalize a smile makeover?

Answer: Most people tend to have some degree of asymmetry. This being said, the dentist may need to modify the size, shape, color and characteristics of the restorations to create the illusion of symmetry within that asymmetric frame. The dentist can mock-up provisional restorations by adding or removing some material in order to give the teeth balance and compliment the facial features, especially if one side of the mouth has more empty dark space than the other. Minimizing the empty dark corridor space on either side of the back teeth and modifying it to create the illusion of symmetry is a critical feature of smile design. If the mouth cants down in one direction so teeth are longer on one side and shorter on the other, we can take steps to balance that and create the visual illusion of symmetry. Laser reshaping of the gum contours or working with a Periodontist, in a team approach, can help to ensure the gum lines appear even and balanced as well. It is a true testament of a successful smile makeover if one cannot readily detect the true imbalance or asymmetry of the patient's facial features.

It is very important to take note and account for a tilted, uneven or asymmetric smile and take the proper photographs, facebow and bite registrations in order to communicate this with the lab ceramist. This is because the asymmetry may be apparent when a person smiles, but not perceived in the impressions or scan of the patient's mouth. The clinical results that we are striving for are directly proportional to the communication skills dentists have with their laboratory. It is suggested that patients undergoing any highly esthetic work or smile makeovers try and arrange to meet with the dental ceramist for a custom shade selection and a more personalized touch.

In an effort to create a more youthful appearance, some examples of how the patient's smile can be designed include having the two upper front teeth just slightly longer than the side front teeth. The canine teeth, which support the corners of the mouth, should be designed to be approximately the same length as the two central front teeth. Rounding the back edges of the incisors can create a softer, more feminine appearance. The curvature of the lower lip can serve as the guide for the ideal smile arc from central incisor to canine.

Question: How can I be certain that the smile designed feels like my smile?

Answer: Proper smile design involves paying close attention to every detail (including esthetics, function and phonetics) before the dental work has even begun. Certain modifications can compensate for someone's asymmetry, and subtle nuances of smile design can help balance and harmonize the smile in order to ultimately lend itself to the creation and illusion of the perfect new smile for that individual. Smile design should be personalized and based upon one's own facial features. The patient's personality and the character of their previous smile may often dictate the need to include different shapes, inclinations and rotations in the design of their teeth and overall smile. Some people may desire or need more prominent canines or more prominent central incisors. Perhaps the lateral incisors may need to be rotated a little to catch the light in just the right way. Each person has his or her own personal preference. Some may desire a more aggressive look, with the edges of all the teeth on the same plane and more sharp angles. Others may desire a softer or more feminine look with rounded back edges and some subtle length differences. There are some who like a more exaggerated positioning of their teeth for a more playful look, with pointier canines and lateral incisors that are more noticeably shorter than their front two teeth. Dentists and ceramists should utilize old photographs and listen carefully to their patients to find out which were the characteristics in their original smile that they liked and disliked. And then, when appropriate, the dentist could give their patients back something in their smile that they once had, in order to make the teeth feel like their own. Proper design is so important, as rejuvenating one's smile with a more youthful, healthier-looking and esthetically enhanced version of what they once had, has the power to inspire their self-confidence and rebuild their self-image.

COSMETIC DENTISTRY

3

(Bonding, Enamel Reshaping, Lumineers, Smile Makeovers, Teeth Whitening, Veneers)

Fun Fact...

Did you know it takes **26** muscles to **smile**?
And **62** muscles to **frown**?

The Importance of a Smile

"A smile increases your face value"

There has been a paradigm shift in dentistry in recent years. A new attitude towards the dentist has emerged, with patients fearing treatment less, and becoming more receptive and excited about doing work that will result in a more esthetically pleasing smile. People used to visit the dentist because they had to, not because they wanted to. Now all of that has changed. People want their teeth whiter, straighter and more beautiful, and they want it done quickly. After all, a smile and a handshake are what create the first impression. A smile and a handshake start every business meeting, every job interview, and leave a lasting impression on a first date. With each passing day, more and more patients are able to recognize how the transformation of a smile can change a life. They know that it will help them or their loved one to land that job, find that special someone, or just give them that extra edge in business and social networking. Individuals are additionally motivated by what they see on television, in the movies and on the pages of magazines. They can appreciate how a beautiful smile can take years off of one's appearance, increase self-confidence and make that person more approachable and distinguished. In fact, often times family members, friends and co-workers have undergone similar smile rejuvenations, which only serve to motivate that individual even more.

Esthetic dentistry is all about creating one's image and inspiring self-confidence. When you are confident with your smile, you are a lot more likely to use it. Patients are a lot more critical of themselves and their appearance these days. With this heightened public awareness, esthetic dentistry is becoming recognized as a necessary treatment for keeping people looking beautiful and healthy. With our minds being educated and our bodies being exercised, what better way is there to communicate how we feel than with a beautiful smile? People simply want to look their best, and once properly educated about their options, will more than likely want to beautify their smile. With in-office tooth whitening and porcelain veneers, all of that is not only possible, but also often done non-invasively and painlessly. In just a couple of visits a smile can be fully transformed. By reshaping the teeth, we create the illusion that the teeth are actually straight and in the proper position. Why should one have to go through life hiding their teeth and being self-conscious about their smile? A reconstructed smile will add confidence and help to create a more youthful appearance. Is the cost a factor? Maybe, but what greater investment could one make than in themselves.

Cosmetic Dentistry

Bonding

Question: What is bonding?

Answer: Bonding uses composite resin to restore chipped or broken teeth, fill in gaps, fix cavities and reshape or recolor your smile.

The same material used for bonding is used for making tooth-colored fillings, which appear more natural. Your dentist applies the resin and sculpts, colors and shapes it to provide a pleasing result. A special light, operating at a specific wavelength, hardens the material, which is then adjusted and polished. Bonding differs from veneers in that bonding can be done within a single visit, while veneers require a dental lab to manufacture the restoration. Additionally, bonded restorations are much less expensive then veneering, since there are no lab costs involved. Bonded restorations are usually very conservative when it comes to reducing tooth structure, and can also be used to protect over exposed root surfaces in order to reduce tooth sensitivity.

Question: How long does bonding last for?

Answer: The answer depends on what the bonding was used for, where in the mouth it was placed, and how well it is cared for. If you place bonding on the biting edge of your front tooth, and like to chew on pen caps or bite your nails, then that bonding is not going to last long. Bonding will usually last for several years before needing to repair it, however, in some areas it can last for many more years with the proper care. Acid reflux and over imbibing in alcohol can weaken the bonded restorations. Teeth grinding can wear down these bonded restorations, but severe teeth grinding will also wear down your own enamel, (the hard, white outer layer of a tooth), along with silver fillings and porcelain restorations. With the proper care, bonding is a wonderful way to restore and improve your smile.

Question: Why do teeth get discolored?

Answer: There are many factors that can affect the color and appearance of your teeth. There are some people who are just born with teeth that are naturally more yellow than others. For example, many blonds and redheads have teeth that tend to be a little bit more on the yellow side due to their genetic makeup. Teeth will also become more yellow and grey with age. This occurs because over many years the enamel starts to wear down, becoming more transparent, and allowing the yellow color of the underlying layer of tooth structure (dentin) to show through. Additionally, there are many other ways that teeth can discolor or stain over time. These can be broken down into two categories: Extrinsic and Intrinsic staining.

- **Extrinsic stains** are the stains that appear on the surface of the teeth as a result of years of consuming coffee, tea, red wine, colas, teriyaki sauce, fruit punch, vegetable juice, highly pigmented foods, and of course, tobacco use. The accumulation of tartar (from the plaque that hardened) will also cause teeth to appear discolored. Superficial extrinsic stains can be readily removed from brushing, flossing and dental cleanings. Deeper stain will need to be bleached out.
- **Intrinsic stains** come from when the actual tooth itself discolors. If someone was given the antibiotic tetracycline during the time when their teeth were forming, chances are they would develop a dark yellowish, brownish banding around the teeth. Excessive ingestion of fluoride can result in fluorosis, which is evident from the white spots that develop on the teeth. Additionally, tooth trauma can result in a color change to the tooth, due to the nerve becoming damaged.

Enamel Reshaping

Question: What is enamel reshaping (enameloplasty)?

Answer: Enamel reshaping is the reshaping and contouring of the enamel (outer layer) of the teeth to remove sharp edges and uneven characteristics of the teeth, and to give the illusion that the teeth are straighter than they really are. This reshaping of the tooth's enamel lends to an improvement of the overall appearance of a smile, correcting the flaws that catch one's eye, such as a tooth that is longer than the others, or an obvious overlapping or rotation of the teeth due to crowding. Enamel reshaping is a conservative process, often combined with some bonding, does not require any anesthesia, and is relatively quick and painless.

Question: Is enamel reshaping harmful to the teeth?

Answer: Enamel reshaping is a very conservative and simple cosmetic procedure, but does remove some of your tooth's enamel, which cannot be replaced. In many respects, enamel reshaping, when combined with teeth whitening and conservative bonding, can be the fastest, least invasive, and least expensive way to have a smile makeover. Granted not everyone is a candidate for this procedure, and many will require a more comprehensive smile makeover to achieve their goals (such as veneers, braces, implants, crown and bridge work, etc.). Often times, enamel reshaping is the intermediary step before committing to a full smile makeover.

Question: Is everyone a candidate for enamel reshaping?

Answer: While many people may be able to benefit from some degree of enamel reshaping, careful case selection is necessary to determine if this procedure is viable for the patient. Many times enamel reshaping in indicated for those people who want to soften the vampire-like points of their canines, or soften and round off sharp, pointy edges, or shorten teeth that appear too long. Very often, as people age, their teeth start to accumulate little chips and wear facets, which eventually cause the teeth to appear less attractive and misshaped. Selective reshaping of the enamel can help to create a more youthful and harmonious smile, but not everyone is a candidate. Individuals with existing restorations or very sensitive teeth may not be good candidates for this. If someone's wear is due to teeth grinding (bruxism), then a night guard appliance would be indicated to prevent further wear, especially after reshaping the enamel. Additionally, if you are planning on having braces, it is recommended not to do any enamel reshaping beforehand, as the areas of the enamel that were modified may become more obvious once the teeth are more perfectly straight. If there are still some minor imperfections or sharp edges after orthodontics, then enamel reshaping may be indicated.

Question: Do teeth become more sensitive after enamel reshaping?

Answer: While most people will have little to no sensitivity from enamel reshaping, there are some whose teeth are very hypersensitive as a result of excessive wear or nerves that are closer to the surface. Your dentist should review your X-rays and assess your level of sensitivity before modifying your enamel. When the outer layer of enamel is reduced, the underlying enamel, once subjected to the oral environment, will function as the new outer layer. Once polished and treated with fluoride, the tooth will have less of a chance of becoming sensitive, and will not become any more prone to developing cavities.

Smile Makeovers

Question: What is a smile makeover?

Answer: Teeth can tell your age...that is, only if you let them. A cosmetic smile makeover can subtract years from your appearance. This smile makeover involves non-surgical modifications, where the smile is broadened, teeth are brightened, and the lips are made to appear fuller. As people get older, their lips usually lose elasticity and become thin, wrinkles develop, and their face begins to show their age.

Smile design takes into account the entire picture, where the lips and gums act as the frame for the esthetically enhanced teeth. Just as different frames complement different paintings, the design and modifications of one's smile are considered on an individual basis. The focus is to improve the entire smile. Fixing just one or two teeth is like renovating one or two houses on a block. It makes everything else look worse. Esthetic dentistry is not patchwork; it is important to concentrate on the entire smile.

The dental profession is currently undergoing an esthetic revolution, where new materials, techniques and equipment have enabled the dental practitioner to produce high quality, highly esthetic restorations that are predictable and minimally invasive. While some people may turn to their plastic surgeon for a face-lift, the cosmetic smile makeover may eliminate the need for that in some cases.

Question: How do you know if someone is a candidate for a smile makeover?

Answer: In order to know if someone is a candidate for a smile makeover the dentist must first evaluate their total face and listen to their expectations. The shape and design of each patient's teeth should be tailored to that individual, because each person's facial contours are different, and these distinct characteristics help to distinguish one's character. The starting point of smile design is determining the facial midline. The midpoint between the two front teeth should line up with the midline of the face. The amount of tooth and gums that are revealed differ from patient to patient depending on phonetics (what their smile looks like when sounding certain letters) and smile position. For example, if you were to draw a line between the corners of the mouth when smiling, you will find that a youthful smile will show 75 - 100% of the front teeth below that line.

Different types of smiles can be created just by altering the planes in which the edges of the teeth line up, and by keeping those edges straight or rounding them off. For example, someone who wants a more aggressive look may have the teeth line up straight across without any soft curves, where as someone who wants a more playful appearance may want the two front teeth slightly longer than the teeth directly next to them, and the canine teeth (two teeth over from the front teeth) would be a little longer and with a more curved point. Just by rounding off the sharp edges of teeth one can create a softer, more feminine appearance. People can also correct that sunken in look where the teeth narrow as they go back by enhancing their smile to fill those dark spaces in the corners of the mouth.

Additionally, esthetic dentistry based upon one's own facial features may dictate the need to include different shapes, inclinations and rotations of teeth. Some people just may need more prominent canines or more prominent centrals. Maybe the laterals need to be rotated to catch the light in just the right way. Old photographs should be used to help find out what characteristics about your original smile you liked and disliked. Then, when appropriate, the dentist can give you some of the characteristics that you liked from the photos you brought in to make the teeth feel more like your own.

Question: Is it realistic to expect that I will look like a model in those magazines after getting having a smile makeover?

Answer: When dentists ask their patients to bring in a photo of a smile that they like, and they bring in a photo of a supermodel and say 'I want to look like this,' is that being realistic? What is it about a model that makes them so photogenic? The reason models photograph so well is because their faces are perfectly symmetrical. If you bisect their faces, you would find that their left and right sides do, in fact, match up. If a dentist took a photograph of all their patients' faces, and then drew a line and bisected it right down the center, they would find that 95% of the time their right side will not match up with their left side. Cosmetic dentists are often taught to make teeth that are symmetrical. Unless their patient has a perfectly symmetric face, they would be doing that patient a disservice in giving them perfectly symmetric teeth. The dental practitioner must take into account the lip curtain, the tilt of the upper jaw, the bone structure, etc., when making the final restorations. Otherwise, they are just placing something completely symmetrical within an asymmetrical frame, which would have the adverse effect of making the teeth stand out.

Question: What steps should I take to prepare for my smile makeover?

Answer: The first thing you should do when planning for a smile makeover is to make sure your dentist takes the time to listen to your desires and to what you like and don't like about your smile. It sounds so simple, but many dentists rush through or ignore this step completely. Your dentist should take digital photographs, perform digital imaging, and create an esthetic wax up that can serve as a template for the temporary restorations. You may wish to meet with the ceramist for a cosmetic consultation and custom shade selection. Feel free to bring in photos of some smiles that you like. The more information you give the ceramist, the more you can guide your dentist to create what will meet or exceed your expectations. It is also recommended to meet with the recommended specialists to help determine if orthodontics or gum reshaping is necessary to enhance your smile even more.

Veneers

Question: What are veneers (aka porcelain veneers, laminates)?

Answer: Veneers are thin pieces of porcelain or resin material that gets bonded (glued) to the front of your teeth. For teeth that are chipped, severely discolored, crowded, spaced, rotated or misshaped in any way, these veneers can create a durable and beautiful smile for many years to come. Veneers are difficult to stain, making them popular for people seeking a perfect smile.

There are two types of veneers:

- Porcelain (indirect) veneers, which must first be created to custom fit your teeth in a dental laboratory and require two visits with your dentist. Porcelain veneers may vary in price from $900-$4,000 per tooth (depending on where you live and the type of dental office you go to) and last from 10 to 15 years or even longer. While more expensive than other alternatives, porcelain veneers usually offer a more precise, realistic color match to your surrounding teeth.
- Composite (direct) veneers, in which composite resins are bonded to your tooth in a single visit. Composite veneers cost significantly less, around $250-$400 per tooth, but usually need to be maintained or replaced sooner than the porcelain version.

Question: What is involved with getting veneers?

Answer: Your dentist must first determine if you are a good candidate for veneers, by taking all the necessary diagnostic records (such as impressions, bite registration, digital photographs, X-rays, etc.). Your original models of your teeth should then be built up in wax to ideal esthetics to see what could be accomplished with the porcelain and how much tooth structure would need to be reduced in order to achieve this ideal wax-up version. Then local anesthetic injections are given, the teeth are prepared, impressions are taken, and temporaries are made. There is an advantage to having temporaries made, which is that is the patient has a chance to take this crude version of their final restorations on a test run to see if they are comfortable when eating, smiling and speaking. If they are not, they have the ability to have them adjusted and modified before the final ones are made. Within a couple of weeks the veneers are bonded onto the prepared teeth, polished and adjusted.

Question: I am over 30 years old and have crowded and crooked front teeth. Is there a way to fix them without having to wear braces?

Answer: Yes, there are a few ways to correct your smile without having to wear braces or retainers. Among your options are Porcelain Veneers, Bonding and Enamel Shaping. In mild cases of crowding, the more conservative approach is Enamel Shaping, which involves modifying the shape of your teeth by removing or contouring enamel (the hard, white outer layer of a tooth) to create the illusion that your teeth are more balanced in their appearance. This process does not require anesthesia, and the results are noticeable immediately. Keep in mind that the removal of enamel is an irreversible process, and may also require additional bonding to enhance the appearance of your teeth. Porcelain Laminate Veneers, in my opinion, are the restoration of choice to correct poorly shaped or slightly crooked teeth for those individuals who do not wish to experience orthodontics. Veneers are thin, custom-made shells made of tooth-colored materials, which are bonded to the prepared teeth to enhance the esthetics of one's smile. This, too, is an irreversible process because a small amount of enamel is usually removed to accommodate the thickness of the porcelain shell. Veneers are used, with tremendous success, for treating gaps and dark spaces between teeth, for teeth that are stained, and for teeth that are worn or eroded at the gum line due to hard tooth brushing. Many of the actors and entertainment personalities who appear to have "picture perfect" teeth have used veneers as a more permanent way to whiten and straighten their teeth. The procedure usually requires 2 or 3 appointments, and the results will make a dramatic difference in the way you look and feel about yourself.

Lumineers

Question: What are Lumineers, and how are they different than traditional porcelain veneers?

Answer: Lumineers (a patented product of the Denmat company) are porcelain veneers are made from an ultra-strong feldspathic porcelain reinforced with leucite crystals. The high strength of the Lumineers allows them to be made contact lens-thin, without increased risk of breakage. The company claims that a dentist can place these veneers without the need for anesthetic injections, extensive tooth preparation, or temporaries. These cases, like traditional veneers cases, can be completed in as few as two visits, but may require less chair time since there is very little tooth preparation, and temporaries are not utilized.

Question: What are the disadvantages of Lumineers?

Answer: Proper case selection is extremely important with Lumineers, as most people are not ideal candidates, without compromising some aspect of the esthetic end product. First, the company claims that you need little to no tooth preparation, which means unless your teeth are very small and inclined inward, the added material of the Lumineers will cause your teeth to appear more bulky. Second, the company claims that their material can be made contact lens thin, so that they won't bulk out the teeth.

However, if they are truly made that thin, and you are trying to change the color of your teeth to a whiter shade, the darker, yellow color of your old teeth will show through (often times in an uneven, blotchy way), causing the end result to fall way short of your esthetic expectations. Third, in order to make dark teeth appear very white, a certain thickness of porcelain would be required. When teeth are already in the ideal position, any additional porcelain would wind up being too bulky and appear more like Chiclets in order to achieve the whiter shade that was selected. Traditional veneers would require enough tooth preparation to allow for the thickness of porcelain to be added to achieve the proper esthetic result. Fourth, the company claims that no anesthesia is indicated since there is little to no tooth preparation. However, since many people have crowded, rotated and protruded teeth, these people may need extensive tooth reduction just to bring their teeth back into the proper alignment. This amount of tooth reduction could become painful without the use of local anesthetic injections. However deceiving their advertising may be, with the right individuals Lumineers can be a great option to have, and can have an excellent end result.

Question: Who is the ideal candidate for Lumineers?

Answer: The ideal candidate for Lumineers is someone who has worn away their teeth, has shorter or smaller teeth inwardly positioned teeth (which can stand to be bulked out a bit), and has spacing between their teeth that they would like to close. Additionally, the ideal candidate would be selecting a shade that is similar to what they are starting with, especially if tooth preparation is not indicated or desired, and the porcelain needs to be thin.

Teeth Whitening (see next chapter) - While teeth whitening is an integral part of cosmetic dentistry, due to the interest and large number of questions it warrants its own chapter.

4

TEETH WHITENING

Fun Fact...

Fifty percent of individuals that were asked say that *the smile* is the first thing they notice about someone.

Show those pearly whites

"A smile and a handshake are the two most important aspects when first meeting someone"

People have become increasingly more preoccupied with health, fitness and beauty. As they diet and exercise their way to a more youthful appearance, they are realizing more and more that one of the hallmarks of appearing youthful is having a bright, beautiful smile. Psychological studies repeatedly confirm that oral and dental beauty is very important to the perception of an individual's confidence and well-being. Smile whitening is no longer a luxury reserved only for the rich and famous. These days, "whiter teeth" is the most popular esthetic request from dental patients, and tooth whitening is a well-tolerated, non-invasive approach to achieving this goal.

Teeth Whitening, though seemingly rather new in the field of dentistry, has actually been around since the 17th century, when people would visit their barbers for a haircut and teeth whitening. Back then barbers would pull teeth and perform teeth whitening by filing down the teeth and applying an acid to them that would cause them to whiten. Of course, this was a fairly painful procedure, harmful to the teeth, and a far cry from where we are today. In 1884, hydrogen peroxide was introduced for teeth bleaching, and the use of high intensity lights were added to accelerate the whitening process starting around 1918. Back then, there were very few cosmetic dentists, and teeth whitening was a procedure that was hardly known. It wasn't until the 1980's that in-office teeth whitening started to become popular, and the early 1990's when over-the-counter whitening products became available thanks to the use of carbamide peroxide. As a result, the dental landscape has since been changed, opening up the doors to hundreds of whitening products and helping to usher in the age of the smile makeover.

Teeth Whitening

Question: What is teeth whitening (teeth bleaching)?

Answer: An estimated ten million Americans will spend a whopping 2 billion dollars on tooth whitening products and services this year to try and achieve that perfect "Hollywood" smile. Tooth whitening is the most common cosmetic service provided by dentists. There are also a growing number of over-the-counter tooth whitening products available as well. Teeth Whitening is a way to reverse the signs of age in teeth, and remove the years of cumulative stain from coffee, wine, soda, teriyaki sauce, tomato sauce, etc. These unsightly stains can be removed quickly, safely, and with minimal discomfort utilizing in-office whitening systems, custom home trays, and over the counter products. You should first have a dental exam to find out which treatment, or combination of treatments is right for you.

Question: Do whitening toothpastes, rinses, flosses and chewing gums actually work?

Answer: Over-the-counter whitening products such as the whitening toothpastes, rinses, flosses and whitening chewing gums are relatively ineffective at best, and some of these whitening pastes can be very abrasive, and actually cause damage to the enamel. Brushing with whitening toothpaste removes the extrinsic stains by mechanical means; little to no change in color actually takes place. The 'whitening' is deceiving on these products, because if it rubs off a little extrinsic stain, does that mean the teeth have been whitened? You need a bleaching agent, such as carbamide peroxide or hydrogen peroxide, in order to intrinsically whiten the teeth. These agents must remain in contact with the enamel for a certain period of time in order to be effective. Even toothpastes that claim to have these agents are not very effective, because they have a mild concentration of peroxide and they are not in contact for long enough duration to make any difference.

Question: Is whitening safe? Does whitening harm your tooth's enamel?

Answer: Tooth bleaching has proven to be a safe and effective way of achieving a more youthful and healthy-looking smile. In fact, the American Dental Association (ADA) has lent its support and approval for enhancing the esthetics of one's smile via in-office and home bleaching, and has given its seal of approval to a number of whitening systems. The safety and effectiveness of this procedure is directly related to the dosage given, the frequency and duration of treatment, the concentration and type of the material used, and the type of tray or system utilized. Like anything, it can be abused, and cause adverse results. During the time that you whiten, the fluoride-rich layer of the enamel is broken down and the teeth become more porous, making them more susceptible to the acids and sugars in your mouth. Within 24-48 hours your tooth's enamel will re-mineralize and build up that protective fluoride-rich layer again. If you become a whitening junkie, and never give your enamel the chance to re-mineralize, then you can cause long-term adverse effects to your teeth.

Question: Which is a better way to whiten your teeth... using an in-office or at-home whitening system?

Answer: In office whitening (i.e. Philip's Zoom! Whitening systems) is a faster alternative for achieving that brighter smile, with a high degree of predictability. This method has been very popular with anyone whose free time is limited or who just wants instant gratification. Many times patients do in-office whitening in combination with custom home trays. The home trays, when used beforehand, can be used to help condition the teeth for more dramatic in-office results. They can also be used for a period of time after an in-office session in order to continue the whitening process, or to help lock in the shade that was achieved. It is recommended to keep your custom trays for periodic touch-ups either before a big event, or to use a couple of times per year to maintain the shade you attained. In-office whitening procedures allow the dentist to whiten their patient's teeth up to 8 shades in about an hour. Some individuals may choose not to wear a custom tray if they are hypersensitive or prone to a gag reflex.

Question: Is it better to wear my home whitening trays during the day or when I sleep at night?

Answer: There are two basic options for home bleaching: daytime and nighttime intervals. Both forms of whitening involve wearing a customized, soft tray, which functions as a reservoir for the whitening gel. Patient compliance is usually better at night, although some people may not be able to tolerate going to sleep with these trays in their mouth. Night use affords the individual maximum benefit from each application because of the longer exposure time and diminished salivary flow. However, occasionally people may need to reduce the duration of their treatment as a result of sensitivity or personal preference. For these individuals, daytime wear is recommended for 1-2 hour intervals of treatment. It is imperative that your dentist professionally supervises this procedure, and that the whitening tray be custom made to ensure a perfect fit.

Question: What is the difference between an over-the-counter whitening strip and pre-formed trays versus a custom tray made in the dental office?

Answer: The importance of a custom-fitted tray cannot be over-emphasized; it allows for maximum patient comfort, reduces side effects, and maximizes efficacy. The over-the-counter versions may be ill-fitting and clumsy, or just may not cover all the desired tooth surfaces that you would want to whiten.

Question: How long does whitening last before I have to do it again?

Answer: With good oral care the procedure's results may last over two years, and recent studies have shown that most patients experience only a one-shade regression after 6 months. Of course, those patients who smoke, drink dark teas and coffee, indulge in red wine and other readily staining foods and beverages are more likely to relapse sooner and require additional whitening sessions. Custom home-tray whitening usually tends to revert less than in-office techniques, but it takes longer to achieve desired results.

Question: Who are the best candidates for teeth whitening?

Answer: If your teeth have been discolored by the natural process of aging, then the prognosis for a beautiful, youthful smile is excellent. Individuals with yellower teeth will typically have a more dramatic result than those with teeth that are greyer in color. Individuals with a more even toned layer of enamel will have a much more predictable result than those with tetracycline stains or white spot formations. The best candidates are those who are whitening their own natural tooth structure. Those patients with restorations of any type, within or covering their tooth structure (i.e. bonding, fillings, veneers, crowns, etc.), must realize that those areas will not whiten. They may choose to still undergo a whitening procedure, but with the understanding that they may require a new restoration in order to match the newly whitened shade.

Question: Do I need to see my dentist first for a cleaning and exam before scheduling a whitening session?

Answer: Yes. It is imperative that one's dentist performs a proper examination and diagnosis, in order to identify abscessed teeth, existing cavities, internal or external resorption, and other pathological problems before bleaching. Your dentist can help you to prevent the "corn-on-the-cob" effect (yellow tooth, white tooth, yellow tooth, etc.), by pointing out which of your teeth have restorations that will not whiten. A cleaning may be indicated to remove the plaque, tartar and extrinsic stains so that the whitening solutions can reach the tooth surface. A full series of X-rays and a detailed dental history should also help to determine if someone is more prone to having sensitive teeth.

Question: How do I prevent my teeth from becoming too white?

Answer: It is extremely difficult to get your teeth "too white" through in-office or home whitening systems. Your teeth have a certain threshold that is difficult to get past with any dentist recommended whitening regimen. Many of these TV personalities and movie stars with the blindingly white smiles got that way not from whitening, but from poorly selecting a shade of porcelain (for their veneers, or crown and bridge work) that was way too white for their skin tones, and as a result it stands out like a sore thumb.

Question: Are there other alternatives to improving my smile other than whitening my teeth?

Answer: Not everyone is a candidate for whitening. Bleaching is not recommended if you have tooth-colored fillings, crowns, caps or bonding in your front teeth, as it will not change the color of these materials, causing them stand out in your newly whitened smile. The best long-term alternative to achieving that picture-perfect white smile is having porcelain veneers, which can be made to become whatever shade you select. This is a much more costly procedure, and usually requires the reduction of some tooth structure (except in certain circumstances). Other alternatives include the use of lighter shade tooth-colored bonded resin materials.

Question: I have whitened my teeth before, but it doesn't look like those actors on TV. What are they doing to get their teeth so white?

Answer: Chances are you are looking at Porcelain Veneers, which are thin, porcelain "shells" that get permanently bonded to the front surface of your tooth. These veneers can eliminate large gaps between teeth, esthetically correct crowded and rotated teeth, and whiten ones smile to their desired shade.

Question: What things should I avoid doing after whitening, and for how long?

Answer: You should avoid anything that can stain a white T-shirt, such as red wine, coffee, tea, cola, teriyaki sauce, tomato sauce, etc. Consume foods and beverages that are bland in color, and closer to room temperature to avoid sensitivity. Within 24 hours from when you completed your last whitening session, the pores of your teeth close, and that fluoride-rich layer will start to build again, protecting the enamel. Once this happens, you may have whatever you wish. Remember that stain is cumulative, and the more bland the diet, the longer the effects will last before you may require another whitening session.

Question: Is there such a thing as over-whitening?

Answer: Yes. There are some whitening junkies or "bleachaholics" who do some form of whitening virtually every day, and don't give their enamel a chance to rest and remineralize. These individuals can damage their nerves and have needed root canals because they have over-bleached. You can also wear away some of the enamel from your teeth and cause them to become more translucent and unnatural. They can become blue or blue-gray in color. Remember, everything in moderation. It is a very safe, gratifying procedure when done as directed by your dentist.

Question: How old does one have to be in order to have whitening performed on them?

Answer: Most dentists will not perform an in-office whitening session on the teeth of someone younger than fourteen years of age. In fact, many prefer to wait until they are closer to sixteen. If some compromise needs to be reached, the dentist may choose to fabricate custom whitening trays and give out a very low concentration gel, or recommend over-the-counter whitening strips or products that are milder and less effective.

Question: Can I still whiten with sensitive teeth? And what can I do to make my teeth more comfortable?

Answer: Most likely, but some determinations must be made first. You should see your dentist to make sure that this sensitivity isn't stemming from some other underlying problem that would need to be addressed more urgently (i.e. a large cavity, fractured tooth, etc.). If there is nothing of an urgent nature, and the sensitivity is due to tooth grinding or clenching, gum recession, exposed root surfaces, etc., then precautions must be taken to make you as comfortable as possible while whitening. For example, the dentist could cover over any exposed root surfaces to protect from the whitening gels. Fluoride toothpastes can be prescribed for use before and after treatments. Desensitizing solutions can be applied either in the office or placed in your custom whitening tray at home, instead of the whitening gel. An over the counter pain medication can be used to help take the edge off the sensitivity if cleared by your dentist.

Question: Does everyone get sensitivity when you whiten your teeth? And how long does the sensitivity last once you get it?

Answer: Some patients may experience sensitivity throughout the treatment; others may not experience any sensitivity at all. Usually any sensitivity one may experience ceases within 24 hours from the termination of treatment. Older teeth have less sensitivity due to the nerves within the tooth becoming less prominent and migrating farther away from the outside surfaces. People with gum recession and root exposure may have more sensitivity due to the bleaching agents coming into contact with those exposed surfaces.

Question: When I used my home whitening trays my gums got irritated? Is that normal?

Answer: Your gums should not become irritated from home whitening treatments. If they do it is most likely due to one of the following reasons: (1) You may have placed too much gel inside the tray causing the excess to extrude onto your gums. You should only need a small teardrop of gel within each tooth reservoir of the tray; do not fill the tray. (2) The trays you were given may not have been properly contoured to the gum line. If this is the case you can ask your dentist to evaluate. (3) The concentration of gel may be too strong for you, in which case you should ask for a lower concentration gel. If the irritation persists after the above has been ruled out, then seek a consultation with your dentist to evaluate for other causes.

Question: After I whitened my teeth, I noticed a bunch of white, blotchy spots all over my teeth…what is that? And what should I do to get rid of them?

Answer: These white spots are due to a decalcification in the enamel. This may happen from a variety of reasons that include the enamel not forming properly during tooth development, and the acid break down of food debris from poor home care. Usually, if someone was not able to clean their teeth well during orthodontic treatment, the food debris would accumulate around the brackets, and the acids would attack that area more to try and break down the food. As a result, once the brackets were removed, white spots would become evident around the area where the brackets used to be.

Question: I have white spots on my teeth…will whitening still work?

Answer: White spots are not removed with bleaching, although they may become less noticeable. If your teeth were dark to begin with, then bleaching may decrease the relative contrast of the white spots on your teeth. If there are any unsightly white spots that remain after whitening, you may choose to trough out those areas and replace it with tooth-colored bonding that blends with the newly lightened shade.

Question: Why do teeth turn yellow?

Answer: Teeth can turn yellow for a variety of reasons, including:

- ❖ Aging (years of cumulative stain and the wear of the outer, white enamel layer of the teeth over time)
- ❖ Heavy consumption foods and beverages which are more likely to stain (including: red wine, dark teas, coffee, vegetable juices, hot chocolate, soy sauce, etc.)
- ❖ Smoking
- ❖ Poor oral hygiene (which creates a thick coat of a yellowing plaque or tartar)
- ❖ Heavy grinding (which can wear away the enamel to reveal the yellower layer of tooth structure beneath)

Please note that the most common cause of this yellowing is due to poor brushing, which builds up this plaque and tartar, which is more likely to hold the stain than the tooth's enamel. Once the teeth are cleaned, the yellow often disappears. Whitening is only effective for brightening the enamel itself, and will not do anything for teeth that are not properly cleaned.

Question: I saw my dentist for an in-office teeth whitening, but my teeth didn't get much lighter. Does this happen to a lot of people? And are there other ways to whiten my teeth?

Answer: Yes, there are a number of people who are more resistant to the effects of teeth whitening. It may happen because their teeth are greyer or perhaps they have tetracycline stained teeth. Whatever the reason, many of these individuals will still whiten quite well utilizing the deep bleaching technique. This technique involves conditioning the teeth on the first visit and slow, time-released exposure during at home wear of the customized whitening trays to create a deep cleansing effect to maximize the penetration of whitening agent into the enamel. After a couple of week of home whitening the patient is then given a full in-office whitening session to bring out the desired effect.

Question: Do toothpastes with color stain your teeth?

Answer: Toothpastes that have color will not stain your teeth generally. However, if you are in the process of undergoing whitening treatments, it is advised to use white toothpaste instead. Teeth can become more porous as a result of bleaching, and are subject to further whitening or staining. Within 24-48 hours after whitening is complete, the enamel regains that protective, fluoride-rich layer, and is not susceptible to the colors within the toothpaste. Additionally, once the toothpaste begins to foam, there is not much color saturating the teeth.

Question: How do I treat and whiten my single dark tooth?

Answer: Treating the single dark tooth can be a challenge. Treatment options include veneers, crowns, bonding or bleaching. Bleaching is the most conservative, but outcomes may vary depending on how dark the tooth is and what caused the discoloration in the first place (i.e. trauma, previous root canal therapy, etc.). Before treating the tooth, it is important to determine what caused the tooth to turn dark and to take the necessary X-rays in order to determine whether the nerve within the tooth is healthy or not.

Bleaching options include:

❖ **The single tooth external bleaching tray** - where the adjacent teeth are cut out so the gel (usually 10-15% carbamide peroxide) only whitens the darker tooth. This tray can be worn for up to 8 weeks in order to bleach the single, dark tooth.

❖ **Internal Bleaching** (only on teeth that have been treated with root canal therapy) – First any material, filler, or residual tissue is removed from inside the chamber. Then whitening and oxidizing agents are placed within that chamber and left for up to 2 weeks and repeated as necessary. Once the desired level of whiteness is achieved, the access hole and chamber are sealed up with a tooth-colored resin. If the tooth does not whiten enough, an opaque white material is used to make the tooth appear even lighter.

❖ **The single tooth internal bleaching tray** – where a bleaching tray is made and the tooth to be bleached is marked. The access hole to the tooth's chamber is left open, after the root canal area is sealed, and the patient is instructed how to fill the area with bleaching gel (usually a more mild concentration such as a 15% carbamide peroxide). This tray is worn for about 1-2 weeks, depending on the bleaching time and the results, before filling up the access area.

❖ **Internal and External Bleaching together** – This is usually the best option for teeth that have been treated with Root Canal Therapy. This type of treatment is accomplished both in the office, at home, or any combination of in-office and at-home treatments.

5

GENERAL DENTISTRY

(Bridges, Crowns/Caps, Dentures, Fillings, Inlays/Onlays, Mouthguard, Occlusion, TMJ)

Fun Fact...

George Washington's dentures were not made from wood. They were made from walrus, hippopotamus, and cow's teeth, as well as elephant tusks.

Dentistry 101 – The Basics

"A canine is man's best friend. So are his incisors, bicuspids and molars."

Dentistry has made some incredible strides from the barber-surgeons of the 17th century to the dental spas of today. Today's Dentists have completed four years of college, four years of dental school and at least one year of residency, compared to the one year of high school required back in 1900. In 1900 about 50% of adults were toothless, compared to a hundred years later when most people have either retained their teeth or replaced them with implants. Some of the most important advances in dentistry over the last century include: the introduction of a local anesthetic in 1905 to make painless dentistry possible; the development of a turbine in dental drills; the development of antibiotics in the mid

1940's to help prevent and control infections; the introduction of fluoride which contributed to a tremendous decline in the incidence of dental cavities; the development of tooth-colored resins and bonding materials; the introduction of dental implants; the introduction of dental lasers for both hard and soft tissues; and the impact of the computer and its related products on dental care. Computer technology has brought about tremendous change in the way dentistry is performed. Prevention has become the mindset of dentists and patients alike, and dentures are becoming a thing of the past. Periodontal disease is being taken more seriously due to the scientific research linking it to various medical conditions such as heart disease and diabetes.

With technology doubling every two years, the future of dentistry is already here... with the scanning of teeth instead of taking messy impressions; using undifferentiated stem cells to grow into an actual tooth with the help of scaffolding matrixes shaped like the tooth it is to replace; integrating 3D digital scans, intraoral cameras and digital X-rays for a more accurate diagnosis; and the ability to create teeth in a day (utilizing an immediately placed implant and a restoration to go over it). Who knows what the next hundred years has in store for us, but for now this chapter answers questions to the most popular aspects of today's general dentistry.

General Dentistry

Bridges

Question: What are bridges?

Answer: Bridges are dental restorations designed to replace the areas where there are one or more missing teeth. There are two basic types of bridges, one is a fixed bridge (which gets bonded or cemented into place) and the other is a removable bridge (which can be taken out and cleaned after meals). The removable bridges are not as secure, and much less desirable than a fixed bridge, although they are much less expensive. Fixed bridges can be made to rest on natural teeth, or on implants, and are usually crowns that are splinted (attached) together. There is also another type of fixed bridge called a "Maryland Bridge," which does not require the use of crowns, but rather utilizes metal or resin wings, coming off the 'fake' tooth, that are splinted or bonded to the inside surface of the adjacent teeth.

Question: How is a fixed bridge attached?

Answer: Just as a regular bridge is built with a strong foundation on both sides and fills in the space between, so does a fixed bridge in dentistry. This fixed bridge rests on strong, healthy teeth on either side of the missing space (called abutments), and fills in the void with 'dummy' teeth (called pontics). The supporting teeth are prepared in the same manner as a crown, where a certain amount of tooth structure gets reduced all around to make room for the material used to fabricate the bridge.

Question: Why would someone need a bridge?

Answer: Reasons for having a bridge include: maintaining your appearance, your dental health, and proper function of your mouth. The loss of a back tooth can cause your cheeks to sink in as you get older, resulting in a much older appearance. Additionally, when you have an empty space, your dental health and mouth's function become compromised in many ways. Your speech can become compromised when you are missing teeth. The adjacent teeth can drift and tilt, causing tooth decay, spacing, gum pockets, and loss of bone. Opposing teeth will tend to slowly erupt out of its socket in attempt to meet up with another tooth. Additionally, if multiple teeth are lost in the back of the mouth, it causes an additional stress on the other teeth, resulting in the enamel to wear down faster. In the case of heavy grinders, missing teeth in the back can cause front teeth to wear down, chip and break, causing their bite to collapse, and slowly break down what is seen when smiling. Missing teeth can affect the way you chew, causing an additional strain on your jaw and TMJ.

Question: How do you clean around a bridge?

Answer: Brushing and flossing must be modified to properly clean around a bridge. There are special shaped brushes and electric brush heads that are designed to clean around a fixed bridge. Waterpiks and rinses are also indicated to help flush out the debris between the teeth. Additionally, there are floss threaders that are designed to thread under the connections of the bridge to allow for a thorough cleaning, along with interproximal brushes and other interdental cleaners that are designed for removing plaque that can accumulate in this area (i.e. rubber tips, plastic picks, etc). Regular dental check-ups are also recommended in order to help keep your bridge clean and your gums healthy.

Crowns/caps

Question: What are crowns (caps)?

Answer: Crowns (also referred to as caps) are dental restorations that surround the prepared tooth structure to help strengthen weakened teeth that have been cracked, broken or decayed. Dentists also use crowns to help restore a tooth's shape and improve chewing function, speech and esthetics. These crowns are made from various types of materials that get bonded or cemented into place. Crowns can be made out of porcelain (or some form of dental ceramic), metal (a gold or other high noble metal alloy), or a combination of both. Since these crowns cover the entire visible potion of the tooth, from the gum level up, they in essence become your tooth's visible surface.

Question: How are crowns made?

Answer: A crown is made in a dental laboratory from the impression or scan that your dentist took of your prepared tooth. Your dentist prepares your tooth by first removing any old, failing restorations, and any weak or decayed areas of tooth structure. Then the core of the tooth is built up with resin type materials that simulate the tooth structure it is replacing. Enough tooth structure is removed all around to allow for the proper thickness of metal and/or porcelain that gets fabricated by the dental lab. On average it takes about 2 weeks for this restoration to be ready for insertion.

Question: When would someone choose a porcelain or all ceramic crown over a traditional porcelain fused to metal crown, and vice versa?

Answer: Porcelain or all ceramic crowns are chosen when esthetics is of paramount importance. These materials can have different shades of porcelain layered together to create a very polychromatic, natural looking tooth with natural translucencies and characteristics that blend better with the teeth surrounding them. Once metal is involved, the dental lab technician would have to place a white opaque material over the metal to try and block out the dark characteristics. As a result of the metal and opaque, the light doesn't get reflected and absorbed as naturally as with a porcelain crown, resulting in a more monochromatic, less natural looking tooth. You can still have good esthetics with porcelain fused to metal crowns, but it may require more tooth preparation to allow for more room for the layering of the porcelain to mask what is underneath. When the patient is a grinder, or requires more strength and stability, it may be recommended to choose a crown that is reinforced with metal, although there are new materials now that are very strong that do not contain any metals (such as Zirconia and Procera crowns).

Dentures

Question: What are dentures?

Answer: Dentures are removable prosthesis or appliances that are designed to replace either all of the teeth (full denture) or some of the missing teeth (partial denture) in the upper or lower jaw. A full denture is only supported by the soft tissues in the mouth and has compromised stability and/or chewing power (unless resting on implants – see Overdenture). Partial dentures are supported in some cases by both the soft tissue and teeth and in other cases just by the teeth, or implants.

Question: Why are dentures needed?

Answer: If someone were to lose some or all of their teeth due to gum disease, tooth decay or injury, a denture would enable that individual to maintain their speech and ability to chew properly. Additionally, dentures can provide support for the lips and cheeks, preventing the face from sagging and appearing older than they really are.

Question: What are the different types of dentures?

Answer: There are various types of dentures, each with a specific purpose or function. These include:

- ❖ **Complete Dentures (Full Dentures)** - This form of denture is made and placed in the mouth of a patient whose gums and bone are fully healed after the teeth have come out. Often times custom made trays will allow for the best impressions to accurately register the anatomy of the area on which the denture will rest. The denture teeth are set in wax, so they can be tried in the mouth and adjusted if necessary. Once the bite, fit and esthetics are acceptable, the denture is processed into a resin base, (sometimes metal can be used), and adjusted until comfortable.
- ❖ **Immediate Dentures** – Immediate dentures are designed so that the patient does not have to be without teeth during the healing period following extractions. The dentist takes the impressions of the patient's mouth before the teeth are removed, and has the denture made without any try–in visit. These often require some adjustments and relining of the denture base to make it fit more comfortably. Since the bone and tissues are constantly remodeling and reshaping after surgery, periodic relines and adjustments are expected, until full healing has taken place, (usually around 6 months). At this time, a new custom fitted complete denture can be made, keeping the immediate one as a spare.
- ❖ **Overdentures** – These types of dentures are a great alternative to help eliminate some of the problems that many

denture-wearers face, including, loose dentures, inability to chew certain foods, and the feeling of being self conscious while wearing dentures. Overdentures are dentures that go over and attach to either natural prepared teeth or implants to form an anchor and add a feeling of security when speaking and eating. Keeping some natural teeth or placing dental implants into the bone beneath the denture helps to maintain the bone level. This prevents the loss of bone normally seen in the jaw after teeth are removed. The teeth involved usually have had root canal therapy, and are cut down to the gum line, with an attachment placed on top that fits into the overdenture. These teeth and implants are the male snap that fits into the female snap of the overdenture. Often times the implants are splinted together into a bar attachment, which is fitted to the inside of the overdenture in such a way that it takes a little effort to snap it out in order to clean it.

❖ **Partial Dentures** – These removable partial dentures have replacement denture teeth that are attached to a gum-colored base and rest on the adjacent teeth by utilizing either metal clasps or a flexible, metal-free alternative. These appliances are very useful as an interim prosthesis while waiting for an implant to be placed and heal. Partial dentures prevent teeth from shifting, acting as a space maintainer, and enable better speech, chewing and esthetics.

Question: How do you care for your dentures?

Answer: Just like natural teeth, dentures should be properly cared for and cleaned after meals. There are brushes that are specifically designed for dentures, but a regular toothbrush may also be used, as long as the bristles are not hard. Ultrasonic cleaners may be used, along with special denture cleaning solutions. Don't let your dentures dry out, or they can lose their shape. Use cool to tepid water because hot water could cause them to warp. Avoid dropping them…they can break! And remember to keep them away from curious children and pets.

Fillings

Question: What are the advantages of having a tooth-colored filling over a silver (amalgam) filling?

Answer: The composite resin (tooth-colored) fillings have come a long way in recent years. Their strength and longevity are now comparable to that of the silver fillings, but with much-enhanced esthetics. The dentist has the capability to match the filling exactly to the shade and color of your tooth so that no one else will ever know you had a cavity. Another advantage of these tooth-colored restorations is that the preparation is relatively conservative. Only decay is removed, and the filling is then bonded to the area that has been prepared. Silver fillings do not have the same bonding capacity, and therefore rely on mechanical retention to hold the filling in place. As a result, good tooth structure is taken away to create the ideal depth and undercuts required to achieve adequate retention. Another advantage of composite restorations is that they are typically less sensitive to hot or cold, as metal tends to conduct temperature more readily.

Question: Is it true that silver fillings may cause health risks?

Answer: Since 1990, when "60 Minutes" ran a story on the alleged risks of dental amalgam (Silver-Mercury fillings), there has been a tremendous amount of media coverage. Reports were made claiming that there have been miraculous "cures" for a variety of medical conditions after these types of restorations are removed, and that dental amalgam is a potential source of mercury toxicity. Mercury constitutes approximately 50% of dental amalgams, and trace amounts of mercury vapor escape in the process of chewing. However, research conducted by the American Dental Academy (ADA), and the scientific community, has concluded that there are no serious health risks associated with silver fillings, and that its removal has not been shown to have any beneficial effects for a patient's specific medical condition. Most dentists utilize mostly the composite resin fillings, not because of health concerns with amalgam, but rather because they are more conservative in terms of reducing tooth structure and because they are much more esthetically pleasing.

Inlays/Onlays

Question: What are inlays and onlays?

Answer: Inlays and onlays are indirect dental restorations that are usually fabricated by a dental lab in order to replace missing tooth structure that resulted from a large area of decay, lost or failing filling, or broken portion of tooth structure. Inlays are restorations that are made to replace the missing tooth structure within the cusps of the tooth, while Onlays are restorations that are designed to extend over and around the missing tooth structure when one or more of the tooth's cusps are compromised. These restorations are like puzzle pieces of tooth structure that get bonded or cemented into place to fill in the missing areas. They are utilized when the amount of missing tooth structure is too large to place a simple filling, but there is enough tooth structure left to avoid having to do a crown. Inlays and Onlays can be made from a tooth-colored ceramic/porcelain material or from a metal such as gold. The tooth-colored inlays and onlays can look so natural and esthetic that it is often difficult to find where the restoration ends and the tooth structure begins.

Question: What is involved in making an inlay or onlay?

Answer: Inlay and onlays, that are fabricated by a dental lab, typically require two appointment visits set about two weeks apart. During the first visit the tooth is prepared (removing any decay, old fillings and weakened, fractured areas), then an impression is taken, and a temporary filling is placed. On the second visit, the temporary filling is removed, and the restoration is tried in and inserted. Local anesthesia is typically given for this procedure, and once it wears away, normal chewing function can resume.

Question: Are there any eating restrictions once I have my inlay or onlay placed?

Answer: It is recommended that you avoid foods that are extra chewy or sticky such as toffees or caramels that will have a lot of upward force on these restorations. Over time, they could break that cement seal, (especially if metal was used as the inlay or onlay material), and cause it to come out. Tooth-colored restorations are bonded, and less likely to come out, but caution should still be taken. Additionally, it is recommended to avoid chewing on hard substances such as ice, hard candies, or certain nuts and seeds, which can exert too much force on the compromised tooth. Gentle test bites should be taken before vigorous chewing to avoid biting down on an un-popped kernel of popcorn or a bone, etc.

Mouthguard

Question: Do I need to get a sports mouthguard?

Answer: Whether you are a professional athlete, a weekend warrior, or just a participant in recreational sport activities, a mouthguard is a must have. Mouthguards are intended to protect not only the teeth and gums, but also your lips, cheeks, tongue, neck, brain, mandible (the lower jaw), and the temporo-mandibular joint (TMJ). Both the American Dental Association (ADA) and the Academy of Sports Dentistry recommend mouthguard use for anyone who engages in sports such as football, softball, racquetball, in-line skating, skateboarding, martial arts, boxing, acrobatics, cycling, equestrian sports, field hockey, ice hockey, handball gymnastics, lacrosse, motor cross, rugby, skiing, shot-put, skydiving, squash, surfing, trampoline, tennis, wrestling, weightlifting and water polo which all run the risk of mouth injuries.

There are several different types of mouthguards, each differing in price and quality. Stock mouthguards are a pre-formed, U-shape piece of rubber or vinyl that you hold between your teeth. It is inexpensive, (and for a very good reason), as the fit is so poor that they are usually not recommended. Mouth-formed mouthguards are available at sporting good stores (as are the stock mouthguards), and they are a step up in quality. There are two types of mouth-formed guards: the boil and bite and the shell-liner. Boil and bite mouthguards are made from a re-formable polymer material that you mold to your mouth by softening the guards in boiling water and then forming it in your mouth. The advantage of this type of guard is that it can be reformed. A shell-liner mouthguard is made by using a stock tray and a resilient liner material that you bite into and wait for it to harden. Unlike the boil and bite, you only have one chance to make it fit. The last class of mouthguards, and certainly the best, is the custom-fit mouthguards that are made by your dentist, impressions will be taken of your mouth, so that they can be made to fit precisely and comfortable. Quality mouthguards are relatively inexpensive, and can prevent injury and the need for costly dental restorative treatments. Naturally, the better quality the mouthguard, the more supportive it will be and the lower the risk of injury. However, the greatest risk of all is to not be wearing a mouthguard.

Night Guard

Question: What are night guards, and why are they important?

Answer: It has been well stated that a smile is one's greatest asset, yet it is not always safeguarded as such. Whether you have all natural teeth, or have just spent a small fortune restoring or cosmetically enhancing your smile, a night guard may be the best way to look after your investment. A night guard (also known as an occlusal splint, a bite guard, and a muscle relaxation appliance) is a device most often recommended as the first line of treatment for bruxism (teeth grinding) and TMD (dysfunction of the TMJ). It is usually worn while you sleep to prevent damaging your teeth by the clenching or grinding associated with either the psychological aspects of stress, one's abnormal bite, a sleep disorder, or a combination of the above. Nightly wear significantly reduces daytime bruxism, because the mouth becomes more sensitized, leading to a heightened awareness whenever the opposing teeth are in contact during abnormal function. A night guard can help reduce your grinding and TMJ troubles by: (1) helping to relax your jaw muscles, which in turn reduce muscle spasms; (2) alleviating your headaches; (3) enabling your jaw to find its best position, since teeth are prevented from locking together; and (4) substituting for your teeth when it comes to wear - it is better to grind the night guard than your own teeth. During the day you should be aware that the only time the teeth should meet is when you chew and when you swallow. All other times think "lips together teeth apart."

Grinding can wear away the surfaces of your teeth causing them to become painful or loose. Although maxillary (upper arch) devices are recommended as the treatment of choice, a lower arch device is indicated when a patient objects to having acrylic visible, or when they have a severe gag reflex with the upper arch device. Quality night guards are relatively inexpensive, and can prevent further wear of your national dentition. They will also help to protect your investment after undergoing a smile makeover. With night guards, it is not enough to simply wear one; they must also be routinely checked and adjusted. Ill devised or poorly adjusted night guards often do not succeed in resolving the problem. Well adjusted night guards (and the acceptable restoration of affected teeth), will allow a patient with bruxism to live a normal life, without significant tooth wear or other dental-related traumas. Remember, we only get one set of adult teeth, so please protect your smile.

Occlusion (bite)

Question: What is occlusion?

Answer: Occlusion (or bite) is how your teeth come together when you close your jaw. Your bite is influenced by three main factors: (1) teeth, (2) nerves and muscles, and (3) bones. Your posture can also influence the way your teeth come together when you close. For example, when you tilt your head back and bite, your teeth will come together differently than when you tilt your head forward and bite. The lower jaw also tends to shift when you are lying down on your side. In an ideal occlusion there is no over bite, under bite or cross bite. All the teeth should come into proper contact when repeatedly opening and closing. An ideal bite or occlusion also has the canine teeth (pointed corner teeth) sliding gently against each other as the jaw slides out to one side, causing the back teeth to not touch.

Question: What are the signs of a poor occlusion or bite?

Answer: Some of the possible signs that your bite may not be right are:

1. Wear facets or indentations on the chewing surfaces of the teeth.
2. Receding gums
3. Erosion or notching of the root surfaces (abfractions)
4. Cracked or fractured teeth
5. Thinning and chipping of the front teeth
6. Pain in the joint and muscles (TMJ pain)
7. Loss of enamel on the chewing surfaces of the back teeth
8. Clenching or grinding of the teeth

Question: What factors can contribute to developing an improper bite or occlusion?

Answer: There are many clues that can indicate early on that a poor occlusion is developing. One clue is when baby teeth are over retained, which can prevent the normal eruption of the adult teeth, causing spacing or drifting of the adjacent teeth. The crowding of lower teeth can indicate that there is an inadequate length of the lower jaw, and a constricted palate can become an issue if not treated with palatal expansion early on. Thumb sucking or abnormal swallowing patterns can result in an anterior open bite.

Question: What are the consequences of having a poor occlusion or bite?

Answer: An improper bite or malocclusion can have detrimental effects on the mouth and the body as a whole. This poor occlusion can cause one to clench and grind their teeth (bruxism), which can result in the loss of enamel, causing teeth to become more sensitive and causing the eventual need for root canal therapy and crowns. When tooth structure is lost, the bite collapses, resulting in the face to develop an older appearance. Grinding can also cause teeth to fracture and can cause mobility of the teeth. When the bite is off, the muscles and joints can become strained, resulting in TMJ problems and jaw pain. When this happens, neck problems and headaches can arise, and one's posture can become affected. Keep in mind that the chewing muscles can exert a lot of force. Normal chewing places about 68-lbs/sq inch of pressure on the back teeth. If you intentionally clench your teeth you may increase that force to about 150-lbs/sq inch. However, an individual who clenches and grinds their teeth subconsciously at night can place up 1200-lbs/sq inch of force.

Question: What do you do to help treat teeth that get translucent at the tip due to lost enamel?

Answer: First you must determine why your teeth are getting more translucent at the top edges. Are they getting translucent as a result of grinding? If so, then a night guard would be indicated to prevent further wear. Are the teeth becoming translucent as a result of some para-functional habit such as nail-biting or chewing on pen caps? Perhaps it is determined that your bite has certain interferences due to crowding, cross-bite, or poorly done restorations, etc. There are times when full mouth reconstruction may become indicated to help open up a collapsed bite to allow for room to repair the translucent areas that resulted from excessive wear. Adding material to translucent areas without making room for it will only result in further grinding or fracture.

TMJ (temporomandibular joint)

Question: What should you do if you are waking up with headaches, and your jaw starts making a popping sound when you open? Is this TMJ related? If so, what causes this, and what can be done to treat it?

Answer: If you are among the millions of people who have been diagnosed with TMJ syndrome, these may be among the symptoms. The TMJ (temporomandibular joint) is a joint that attaches the lower jaw to your skull. The symptoms described may be a result of the TMJ not functioning properly, due to one or more of the following having been adversely affected: your chewing muscles, joints, ligaments or surrounding bones. It is difficult to pinpoint the exact cause of one's TMJ syndrome, although it is often related to stress. It also may be the result of a traumatic accident or a disease such as arthritis.

Question: What are the most common causes of TMJ discomfort?

Answer: The most common causes of TMJ are clenching and grinding, which can tire and strain the chewing muscles, causing them to go into spasm and cause pain. An improper bite can also result in TMJ dysfunction. Among the symptoms are: headaches (usually upon awakening), tenderness or fatigue of the jaw muscles, earaches, and pain or difficulty when chewing, yawning or opening your mouth wide. Clicking or popping sounds are very common signs, and in some extreme cases, the jaw can actually get stuck in the open or closed position.

Most cases of TMJ disorders can be treated conservatively and successfully. Only a small number of cases require surgical correction, usually with those individuals who have suffered a traumatic injury. The first step is to eliminate the pain and muscle spasms. In mild cases, this can be done with moist heat packs, a non-chewy diet, and muscle relaxants (if necessary). It is also important not to try to test the degree of pain by opening and closing, but rather try to rest the TMJ and give it time to heal.

The next step would be to try and become aware of the potential sources of stress and tension that could lead to clenching and grinding. A conservative therapeutic device that may work well for you is a corrective bite plate, (made by your dentist), that will help to relax the muscles, thus preventing headaches, pain and spasm. Selective filing of an uneven bite to correct the "high" spots is a final attempt to treat TMJ conservatively, because the removal of tooth structure is an irreversible process.

Question: I was having tooth pain after a tooth chipped on the left side. Now the pain moved to the right side, along with jaw pain and extreme headaches. Is this a tooth issue or a neurological issue?

Answer: What most likely happened was that you traumatized or fractured a part of that tooth on the left side, causing you to consciously or subconsciously avoid chewing on that side. As a result of chewing everything on the right side, you are putting a lot of strain on the right TMJ (temporomandibular joint), resulting in jaw pain and headaches. Once you address the problem on the left side, you should be able to even out your chewing and allow for this discomfort to go away.

Myth vs. Fact

Myth: Gum chewing is bad for your teeth.

Fact: Chewing sugar-free gum can actually be good for your teeth. It helps to neutralize the acids in your mouth, and lift out the food debris that gets trapped in the pits and grooves of your teeth. When you cannot get to a toothbrush, gum chewing is a nice alternative after having a meal or snack. It is the sugared gums that you should avoid at all costs. Additionally, you should limit the length of time you chew gum for because lengthy chewing can aggravate your TMJ and cause discomfort and strain on that joint.

6

IMPLANT DENTISTRY

Fun Fact...

In the dark ages it was believed that a
person could regrow a lost tooth simply
by obtaining and possessing a tooth from
someone else – preferably a hanged criminal.
We've come a very long way since then.

We can rebuild you better and stronger...

"With implants, teeth can appear to last a lifetime"

Dental implants have come a very long way since their first introduction 2,000 years ago when people crudely tried to replace their lost teeth with animal teeth or with teeth purchased from the poor and from slaves. For centuries following, it just seemed easier and a lot less uncomfortable to wear false teeth or simply go without them. To put things in perspective, in the early 1900's, the average lifespan was 47 years old, and 50 percent of adults were toothless back then. With people becoming more esthetically self-conscious and living a lot longer, the need for predictable and comfortable tooth replacement has become increasingly more important.

Starting in the 1950's, dentists began experimenting with blade implants, which were flat metal pieces that were attached to the bone, but never actually integrated with it. They had a 50 percent success rate, and when they failed, they often caused a lot of damage to the surrounding area. In the mid 1960's it was discovered that titanium could be used to fuse to bone and support replacement teeth. Initially, implants were only placed in the front part of the lower jaw where the bone was denser and the nerves were not in the way. In the 1980s, the technology progressed to the point where these titanium implants could be placed in all areas of the mouth for those with enough bone to support it. Eventually, bone grafting procedures made it possible for implants to be placed in the mouths of those who were not previously candidates for implants.

The size, shape, strength and design of the implants are continually improving each year, with success rates between 95-99 percent depending on the area being worked on. The techniques for placing these implants have also improved, as some people are candidates for placing implants and their replacement teeth in the same day. These implants are quickly displacing the need for wearing removable dentures or fixed dental bridges. What does the future hold in this area of dentistry? Who knows? Within a short period of time dentists may possibly be implanting actual tooth buds harvested from stem cells that grow to become the tooth that needs to be replaced.

Implants

Question: What is implant dentistry?

Answer: The introduction of implant dentistry has laid the foundation for a new level of care and service that accomplishes today what was thought impossible only a few years ago. It is the most advanced therapy available to replace missing or lost teeth. Dental implants not only enable one to regain their confidence and psychologically be able to enjoy an active lifestyle, but they can improve your smile, help you to once again enjoy chewing all the foods you like, and help to restore your facial structure and youthful appearance. Implant dentistry and bone regeneration are among the recent miracles of modern medicine. Their impact on the field of dentistry ranks up there with the introduction of the local anesthetic Novocain (developed in 1904), and the air-driven turbine drill (introduced in1957). With adequate time and proper planning great things can now be accomplished.

Question: What are dental implants?

Answer: Implants are metal posts (usually titanium) that are surgically placed beneath your gums to act as artificial tooth roots once they have become integrated with the surrounding bone. These implants offer stable support to artificial teeth, whether in the form of a single crown, a fixed bridge or beneath a removable denture. A conventional fixed bridge still remains an excellent treatment option. However, many individuals who have lost or who will be losing a single tooth may be hesitant to grind down their intact adjacent teeth, especially when the adjacent teeth are free of cavities or restorations. For these individuals, a single tooth dental implant may be the ideal option.

Question: Is everyone a candidate for implants?

Answer: As with any medical or dental procedure, the placement of implants may have a compromised success rate in certain individuals. Some of the reasons to exclude dental implants as a treatment option include: insufficient bone quantity, poor bone quality, inadequate amounts of space between your upper and lower teeth, vital anatomical structure in close proximity to the proposed implant site, unrealistic expectations about the esthetic outcome, or a still growing mouth and face. Certain chronic diseases such as diabetes, osteoporosis or chronic sinus troubles can have the potential to interfere with the integration of bone to these implants. Individuals who smoke regularly will usually have a poorer prognosis for the implants in the long run. However with proper treatment planning, placement selection, and by utilizing the appropriate style of implant, the level of success has been tremendous. To find out if implants are the right choice for you, your dentist will need to evaluate your health history, take impressions of your mouth for planning models, and take the necessary dental X-rays. Your dentist will most likely refer you to have a CAT scan performed to help establish the quality and quantity of your bone, along with determining the best placement and the number of implants that will be required for long-term success.

Question: Are implants more successful in different areas of the mouth?

Answer: Yes. Different areas of the mouth typically have different qualities of bone. For example, the front segment of the lower jaw has the densest bone, while the back portion of the upper jaw usually has bone that is softer and more porous. Implants will have a better chance of success in an area of denser bone. If it is discovered that you do not have enough bone in certain areas, do not yet give up hope. Recent studies have proven that implants can be quite successful in bone that has been augmented by either natural or synthetic bone grafts. The degree to which new bone will form within the grafted site differs from one individual to another depending on the type of graft used and the overall health of the patient.

Question: How do you care for implants?

Answer: The long term success of implants is, in part, determined by meticulous oral hygiene and regular dental visits. Although you cannot get cavities in implants or periodontal disease, it is possible to develop what is called peri-implantitis, which is inflammation of the tissues around the implants. To prevent this, keep brushing and flossing as you normally would your own teeth, and don't forget to schedule your regular check-ups.

Question: Are these implant procedures painful?

Answer: These procedures are performed without discomfort, under the utilization of local anesthesia or local anesthesia with I.V. Sedation. Occasionally general anesthesia may be used depending on the individual and their medical history. Post-operatively there may be mild to moderate discomfort and some swelling, but nothing that can't be controlled with the assistance of an oral analgesic that your doctor will prescribe.

Question: Am I a candidate for a single tooth immediate implant?

Answer: Another topic to be of considerable interest for discussion is whether or not one is a candidate for placing a single tooth implant in a fresh extraction site (tooth socket). Dentists regularly wait for a period of 6 months after extracting a tooth before they place an implant. However, this delays treatment and may leave the residual bony ridge too thin for implant placement. A thin or resorbed bony ridge is of primary concern in areas where the esthetics of one's smile is in jeopardy of being compromised. This compromised quantity of bone could lead to cosmetic defects such as the loss of the surrounding gum tissue. It is believed that bone growth may actually be greatest after a tooth is removed. Single tooth immediate implant placement (according to a 1997 regeneration report in the *Journal of Practical Periodontics and Aesthetic Dentistry*) is indicated in the following cases: (1) teeth that are lost by trauma, (2) teeth that are condemned due to fracture, (3) residual baby teeth with root resorption, and (4) teeth with root canal failure. The disadvantage of immediate placement is that placing an implant in a fresh extraction site does not provide optimum initial bone-to-implant contact. As a result, the usual waiting period for the implant to integrate with the bone may have to be extended by about 2 months. Depending on what implant system is used, this usual waiting period generally take anywhere from 2 to 6 months before the implant can be restored with a crown. The immediate implant procedure has survived 10 years of clinical scrutiny and has a proven success rate that is close to those experienced in an intact toothless site. Keep in mind, however, that this procedure is not generic; it is only presently indicated for those individuals who satisfy the aforementioned criteria.

Myth vs. Fact

Myth: If I lose a tooth in the back of the mouth it is not a big deal, because no one sees it anyway.

Fact: Many people prioritize their dental health by taking care of the teeth they can see when they smile and put off care for the teeth they do not see. A number of patients will choose to spend their money whitening their front teeth, instead of putting those funds towards restoring a compromised back tooth. When that back tooth fails, and needs to be removed, the space often gets left there without a bridge or an implant to help fill in the space. Empty spaces in the back are a big deal! When you have an empty space, the adjacent teeth can drift and tilt, causing spacing, gum pockets, and loss of bone. Opposing teeth will tend to slowly erupt out of its socket in attempt to meet up with another tooth.

Additionally, if multiple teeth are lost in the back of the mouth, it causes an additional stress on the other teeth, resulting in the enamel to wear faster. In the case of heavy grinders, missing teeth in the back can cause front teeth to wear, chip and break, causing their bite to collapse, and slowly break down what is seen when smiling.

7

PERIODONTICS (GUM DISEASE)

Dental Fact...

Most tooth loss in people over age
35 is from Periodontal Disease.

Periodontal Disease: What you need to know to keep your teeth for a lifetime

*"If the teeth are the star
performers, the gums and bone
are the supporting cast that helps
to keep your production going
for many years to come"*

Periodontal disease (gum disease) is a slowly progressing, silent disease that affects the supporting structures of the teeth, (such as the gums and surrounding bone), and is more responsible for tooth loss than dental cavities. Often times it is not painful, and goes unnoticed until the dentist or hygienist makes you aware of the problem. More than 75 percent of the population has some form of gum disease, and we are learning more and more about the links between gum disease and other conditions such as heart disease and diabetes. As dentists start to check for signs of periodontal disease more routinely, and as patients become more educated about what they can do to address and prevent this disease, we can begin to take the necessary steps to control this often neglected facet of dentistry.

Periodontics (Gum Disease)

Question: Who is a periodontist?

Answer: A periodontist (the gum specialist) is a dentist who specializes in the prevention, diagnosis and treatment of periodontal disease and in the placement of dental implants. Periodontists receive extensive training in these areas, including three additional years of education beyond dental school. Periodontists are familiar with the latest techniques for diagnosing and treating periodontal disease. In addition, they can perform cosmetic periodontal procedures to help you achieve the smile you desire. Often, dentists refer their patients to a periodontist when their periodontal disease is more advanced.

Question: What is periodontal disease?

Answer: Periodontal (gum) disease, including gingivitis and periodontitis, are serious infections that, left untreated, can lead to tooth loss. The word *periodontal* literally means "around the tooth." Periodontal disease is a chronic bacterial infection that affects the gums and bone supporting the teeth. Periodontal disease can affect one tooth or many teeth. It begins when the bacteria in plaque (the sticky, colorless film that constantly forms on your teeth) causes the gums to become inflamed.

Question: What is gingivitis?

Answer: Gingivitis is the mildest form of periodontal disease. It causes the gums to become red, swollen, and bleed easily. There is usually little or no discomfort at this stage. Gingivitis is often caused by inadequate oral hygiene. Gingivitis is reversible with professional treatment and good oral home care.

Question: How do I know if I have early gum disease (gingivitis) or late stage gum disease (periodontitis)?

Answer: In the early stages of gum disease, the plaque that remains around the teeth harden into calculus (tartar). As plaque and calculus continue to build up, the gums begin to recede (pull away) from the teeth, and pockets form between the teeth and gums. At this stage, with treatment, it is fully reversible. As gum disease progresses, the gums recede further, destroying more bone and the periodontal ligament that surround the roots. The affected teeth become loose and may need to be extracted. Routine check-ups and periodic measuring of the pockets around the teeth are necessary to monitor and prevent gum disease from progressing.

Question: What is periodontitis?

Answer: Untreated gingivitis can advance to periodontitis. With time, plaque can spread and grow below the gum line. Toxins produced by the bacteria in plaque can irritate the gums, and stimulate a chronic inflammatory response in which the body, in essence, turns on itself and the tissues and bone that support the teeth are broken down and destroyed. Gums separate from the teeth, forming pockets (spaces between the teeth and gums) that become infected. As the disease progresses, the pockets deepen and more gum tissue and bone are destroyed. Often this destructive process has very mild symptoms. Eventually, teeth can become loose and may have to be removed.

Question: What are the different forms of periodontitis?

Answer: There are many forms of periodontitis. The most common ones include the following:

- ❖ **Acute periodontitis** occurs in patients who are otherwise clinically healthy. Common features include rapid attachment loss and bone destruction.
- ❖ **Chronic periodontitis** results in inflammation within the supporting tissues of the teeth, progressive attachment and

bone loss. This is the most frequently occurring form of periodontitis and is characterized by pocket formation and/or recession of the gums. It is prevalent in adults, but can occur at any age. Progression of attachment loss usually occurs slowly, but periods of rapid progression can occur.

❖ **Periodontitis as a manifestation of systemic diseases** often begins at a young age. Systemic conditions such as heart disease, respiratory disease, and diabetes are associated with this form of periodontitis.

❖ **Necrotizing periodontal disease** is an infection characterized by necrosis of gingival tissues, periodontal ligament and alveolar bone. These lesions are most commonly observed in individuals with systemic conditions such as HIV infection, malnutrition and immunosuppression.

Question: How do I know if I have periodontal disease?

Answer: Periodontal disease is often painless and develops slowly and progressively. Sometimes it may develop quite rapidly. Unless you see your dentist for regular checkups, you may not realize you have periodontal disease until your gums and bone have been severely damaged to the point of tooth loss. Periodontal disease can occur at any age. In fact, more than half of all people over age 18 show signs of at least the early stages of some type of periodontal disease. Gingivitis is the earliest stage of periodontal disease and affects only the gum tissue. At this stage, it is reversible. If not treated, it could lead to periodontitis, potentially damaging bone and other supporting structures. Such damage can result in loosened teeth.

Question: What can I expect the first time I have a periodontal evaluation by my dentist or periodontist?

Answer: During your first visit, your dentist or periodontist will review your complete medical and dental history with you. It's extremely important for your periodontist to know if you are taking any medications or being treated for any condition that can affect your periodontal care. You will be given a complete oral and periodontal exam. Your periodontist will examine your gums, check to see if there is any gum line recession, assess how your teeth fit together when you bite and check to see if you have any loose teeth. Your periodontist will also take a small measuring instrument and place it between your teeth and gums to determine the depth of those spaces, known as periodontal pockets. This helps your periodontist assess the health of your gums. Radiographs (X-rays) may be used to show the bone levels between your teeth to check for possible bone loss.

Question: Is it true that there is a link between periodontal (gum) disease and heart disease?

Answer: Studies show periodontal disease can contribute to increased risk of heart attack and stroke. According to some studies, periodontal disease (which affects the bone and tissue surrounding your teeth) has proven to be a stronger risk factor than any of the other conditions usually linked to heart disease (i.e., hypertension, high cholesterol, age and gender). Researchers have concluded that the bacteria found in plaque (the primary etiological factor causing periodontal disease) is clearly linked to coronary disease. People with periodontal disease are up to two times as likely to suffer a fatal heart attack and nearly three times more likely to suffer a stroke as those individuals without this disease.

Question: What can I do to prevent periodontal disease?

Answer: Keep your teeth clean by brushing with fluoridated toothpaste at least twice daily. Use dental floss and mouth rinse. Eat a balanced diet for good general health to secure the proper amount of nutrients to build your mouth's resistance to the infection caused by bacterial plaque. Visit your dentist at least every six months for a checkup; making sure that a thorough periodontal exam is performed. Avoid other risk factors such as smoking and chewing tobacco, both of which have a detrimental effect on the severity of periodontal disease. Systemic diseases such as AIDS or diabetes can lower the oral tissue's resistance to infection, making periodontal disease more severe. Review your medical history with your dentist. Many of the medications or therapeutic drugs that you may be taking can decrease your salivary flow and adversely affect your teeth and gums.

Question: What is the link between periodontal disease and diabetes?

Answer: More and more studies are showing a link between the mouth and the rest of the body regarding the spreading of infections. Over 400 different types of bacteria can exist in the human mouth. Many of them thrive in sugars, including glucose, the sugar linked to diabetes. Persons with diabetes have greater than normal risk of gingivitis (inflammation and bleeding of the gums) and periodontal disease, the condition that causes millions to lose their teeth. Like any infection, gum disease can make controlling the blood-sugar level very difficult. Diabetes causes the blood vessels to thicken, in turn slowing the flow of nutrients and the removal of harmful wastes. The result is a weakening of the resistance of the gums and bone tissue to the spread of infection. Researchers have found that diabetes predisposes a patient to periodontal disease. Moreover, recent evidence strongly suggests periodontitis can worsen the severity of one's diabetic condition.

Many diabetic patients with severe cases of periodontal disease struggle to maintain their normal blood-sugar levels, and as a result their need for insulin increases. Infections originating in the mouth can easily spread, and may enter the bloodstream. In cases of severe gingivitis and periodontal disease even the simple act of brushing or flossing can introduce bacteria into the bloodstream, aggravating health troubles in other areas of the body. Experts expect that treatment of periodontal disease may diminish fluctuations of blood-sugar levels, along with a decreased risk of diabetic retinopathy and the associated risk of damage to the arteries.

People with diabetes are also at risk for developing thrush, a yeast infection in the mouth that causes white spots on the tongue. This infection thrives on high glucose levels in saliva. Another oral manifestation found in uncontrolled or undetected diabetics is dry mouth (xerostomia), an ailment that may result in halitosis (bad breath). Smokers are five times more likely to develop gum disease. A smoker with diabetes aged 45 or older is 20 times more likely to get severe gum disease.

Question: What precautions should I take when I see my dentist if I have diabetes?

Answer: If you have diabetes, make certain you inform your dentist and book a visit for an examination and cleaning at least every six months. You should schedule your dental appointments for about an hour and a half after breakfast and after you have taken your diabetes medication. Try to arrange shorter visits, preferably in the morning.

Question: Is there a relationship between tobacco use and periodontal disease (smoking, tobacco, gum disease, periodontal disease?

Answer: Studies have shown that tobacco use may be one of the most significant risk factors in the development and progression of periodontal disease. Smokers are much more likely than non-smokers to have calculus form on their teeth, have deeper pockets between the teeth and gums and lose more of the bone and tissue that support the teeth.

Question: Is it normal for my gums to bleed when I brush my teeth?

Answer: No, it is not normal for your gums to bleed when you brush. Bleeding gums are one of the signs of gum disease. It is an indication of the beginning of the destructive process involving the supporting tissue around the tooth or possibly some serious underlying systemic problems. The bacteria, which cause gingivitis (inflammation of the gums), can turn into tartar buildup, irritate your gums and lead to bleeding. If left unchecked, gingivitis can lead to a more serious form of gum disease called periodontitis. This long-term infection can eventually cause loss of your teeth.

Question: What does it mean to have receding gums? What can be done for this?

Answer: There are a few reasons why one might develop receding gums. One way is by using an improper brushing technique (i.e. brushing in an up and down or circular motion with a manual brush, rather than with small, vibratory strokes on a 45 degree angle). Another reason involves using a brush that has harder bristles or that is frayed and overdue for being replaced, which can traumatize the gums. Sometimes there may be high muscle attachments, (attaching the inner part of the lips to the gums), which pull down on the gum tissue over time as one speaks, smiles, eats, etc. Additionally, gums can recede as a result of periodontal disease, due to the bone loss beneath.

While the gum tissue may not grow back on its own, there are a few things one can do to help prevent gums from receding further. Among the suggestions are:

❖ Use an electric brush
❖ If using a manual brush make sure to use soft bristles
❖ Use the proper brushing and flossing technique
❖ Consider reattaching the muscle attachments so that they are not pulling down on the gums (frenectomy).
❖ See your dental provider frequently to avoid developing periodontal disease (gum disease)

Question: What are the warning signs of gum disease (periodontal disease)?

Answer: There are a number of warning signs of gum disease, which include the following:

❖ Red, swollen or tender gums or other pain in your mouth
❖ Bleeding while brushing, flossing, or eating hard food
❖ Gums that are receding or pulling away from the teeth, causing the teeth to look longer than before
❖ Loose or separating teeth

❖ Pus between your gums and teeth
❖ Sores in your mouth
❖ Persistent bad breath
❖ A change in the way your teeth fit together when you bite
❖ A change in the fit of partial dentures

Question: What does it mean to have pockets when you check for gum disease?

Answer: Your bone and gum tissue should fit snugly around your teeth like a turtleneck around your neck. When you have periodontal disease, this supporting tissue and bone is destroyed, forming "pockets" around the teeth. Over time, these pockets become deeper, providing a larger space in which bacteria can live. As bacteria develop around the teeth, they can accumulate and advance under the gum tissue. These deep pockets collect even more bacteria, resulting in further bone and tissue loss. Eventually, if too much bone is lost, the teeth will need to be extracted.

Question: Could my periodontal disease be genetic?

Answer: Research proves that up to 30% of the population may be genetically susceptible to gum disease. Despite aggressive oral care habits, these people may be 6 times more likely to develop periodontal disease. Identifying these people with a genetic test before they even show signs of the disease and getting them into early interceptive treatment may help them keep their teeth for a lifetime.

Question: What can I do to avoid periodontal disease?

Answer: To keep your teeth for a lifetime, you must remove the plaque from your teeth and gums every day with proper brushing and flossing. Regular dental visits are also important. Daily cleaning will help keep tartar formation to a minimum, but it won't completely prevent it. A professional cleaning at least twice a year is necessary to remove tartar from places your toothbrush and floss can't reach or may have missed.

Question: What kind of oral care products should I use to prevent against gum disease?

Answer: Begin with the right equipment – use a soft bristled toothbrush that allows you to reach every surface of each tooth. If the bristles on your toothbrush are bent or frayed, buy a new one. A worn-out brush will not clean your teeth properly. In addition to manual toothbrushes, your choices include electric toothbrushes. These are safe and very effective when used properly. Oral irrigators (water spraying devices) are a great adjunct, but will not remove plaque from your teeth unless they are used in conjunction with brushing and flossing. Another aid is the rubber tip, often found on the handle end of a toothbrush used to massage the gums after brushing and flossing. Other options include interproximal toothbrushes (tiny brushes that clean plaque between teeth) and interdental cleaners (small sticks or picks that remove plaque between teeth). If used improperly, these dental aids can injure the gums, so it is important to discuss proper use with your periodontist. Prebrushing rinses, such as Plax, or post brushing rinses and fluoride rinses or treatments are encouraged. Of course dental floss, when used properly, will help to prevent against cavities and gum disease. It is also recommended to use a tongue scraper to clean the posterior third of your tongue to prevent against oral malodor.

Question: If I neglected my teeth for years, am I able to get them back to a completely healthy state?

Answer: If your teeth have been neglected for years, chances are you have already done some irreversible damage. Gum disease can cause a loss of bone support, which will not grow back once the mouth returns to a completely healthy state. The gum recession that follows the bone loss will remain evident, unless you are a candidate for certain gum and bone grafting procedures. The good news is that you can arrest bone loss and gum recession by taking perfect care of them. In other words, while you may not get back to where you started, you can prevent further damage from occurring.

Teeth that are broken and/or have decay can often be restored and brought back to proper function and esthetics. Teeth that are beyond repair can be removed and replaced with implants and bridge work to regain chewing surfaces and enhance the mouth's esthetics. Take one step at a time, and once you are at a completely healthy state, make sure to see your dentist regularly to maintain.

Question: My gums bleed in the same spot every time I brush my teeth. What can be done to help this?

Answer: Chances are, if your gums are bleeding in the same spot every time you brush, there is an underlying reason for it. It may be that there is a piece of tartar deep within the pocket surrounding the tooth and it needs to be removed to allow for the gums to reattach to the tooth and become healthy once more. Perhaps there is an overhang of a filling or a piece of cement wedged beneath the gums. Bleeding is a sign of inflammation, and inflammation is usually brought about by some outside stimulus such as a trapped piece of popcorn, a seed, a string of the floss, or simply just the bacteria from plaque and tartar. Remove the stimulus; maintain the area and the bleeding will disappear.

Myth vs. Fact

Myth: Bleeding gums are normal.

Fact: Bleeding gums are NOT normal. It is a sign that something is wrong and that there is some form of gum disease present. Bleeding results from inflammation of the gums (gingivitis), due primarily from inadequate removal of plaque from the teeth at the gum line. If this plaque is not removed (through regular brushing and routine dental care), it will harden into a substance called tartar, and eventually lead to increased bleeding and gum and bone recession (periodontal disease). In some cases, chronic bleeding can be due to a pre-existing medical condition or blood disorder. Because it is usually painless, many people think it is normal, but it is not. If your gums bleed when you brush, it might be that you are brushing too hard or using a very hard brush and cutting the gums, but that is not likely because it would be painful. It is most probable that you are not brushing effectively. Daily removal of bacterial plaque, along with regular periodontal cleanings will enable you to have a healthy mouth with healthy teeth and gums.

8

ENDODONTICS (ROOT CANAL)

Fun Fact...

During the Middle Ages in Germany, you would have been advised to kiss a donkey in order to relieve your toothache.

Root Canals: Understanding the root of the problem and its procedures

"Just the words 'Root Canal' seem to strike a nerve with a lot of people"

Root canal therapy (endodontics) has come a very long way since its start in the 17th century. Imagine having the nerve of your tooth removed with a filed down watch spring without any anesthesia. Back in 1838 this was thought to be innovative, along with the use of arsenic and heated instruments to cauterize the nerves. No wonder why root canals got such a bad reputation. Since then, there have been numerous advances and developments, such as safe and effective local anesthetics after 1910, dental X-rays, (which became commercially available in 1919 for dentists), and much more high tech instruments and medicaments. Additionally, lab research and clinical evidence helped to shift the mindset in the early 1950's from extracting all teeth whose nerves were no longer alive, (since it was previously thought to be the source of numerous diseases and ailments), to saving the teeth by performing root canal therapy.

The aim of endodontics has always been to relieve pain and preserve teeth. Today, patients can feel comfortable knowing that root canal procedures are reliable, safe, and no more uncomfortable than placing a filling, due to the advances in technology and local anesthetics. Root canal treatment tends to have a very high success rate, and most can last for a lifetime.

Endodontics (Root Canal)

Question: What is an endodontist?

Answer: An endodontist is a dental specialist dedicated to root canal treatment, relieving oral and facial pain, and saving natural teeth. Many endodontists use a microscope that allows them to see the space within the tooth with great magnification and clarity. The microscope enables them to locate tough-to-find nerve canals within the tooth so they can more thoroughly clean them, and to see cracks that would otherwise go undiagnosed. The microscope is an advanced piece of equipment that far exceeds the capability of dental loupes (binocular-like magnifiers worn by many dentists). While many dental practitioners feel comfortable performing root canal procedures on their patients, if they feel that a root canal procedure is very complicated, or out of their comfort zone, they will refer their patient to an endodontist.

Question: What is root canal therapy?

Answer: Root canal therapy is when the endodontist removes the inflamed or infected pulp (nerve), carefully cleans and shapes the nerve canals of the tooth's root and then seals the prepared space. Most treatment is performed in one or two appointments ranging from 30-90 minutes each (depending on the number of canals). Once treatment is completed, you may be instructed to return to your dentist for a more permanent restoration. This restoration of the tooth is an important part of treatment because it seals the cleaned canals from the oral environment, protects the tooth and restores it to function.

Question: Why would someone need a root canal?

Answer: Root canal therapy (endodontic treatment) is necessary when the nerve (pulp) becomes inflamed or infected. The most common reasons for inflammation or infection are deep cavities, repeated dental procedures, cracks or chips. Trauma can also cause inflammation and often shows up as discoloration of the tooth. If pulp inflammation or infection is left untreated, it can cause pain or lead to an abscess.

Question: What are the signs and symptoms that root canal therapy is indicated?

Answer: Indications for treatment include prolonged sensitivity to heat or cold, spontaneous pain, discoloration of the tooth, and swelling or tenderness of the tooth or adjacent gums. Transient sensitivity to cold may just be due to exposed root surfaces or heavy teeth grinding. If the cold sensation lingers, and radiates up to give you a headache, chances are there has been irreversible damage to the nerve. Sensitivity to heat is usually a clear indication that there is some nerve damage present. Sometimes there are no symptoms, and diagnosis is made from a routine X-ray. Other times, root canal treatment is recommended as a result of the bacteria from the decay extending into the nerve (pulp) of the tooth; this would be seen by the dentist during their examination of the tooth.

Question: What is the pulp?

Answer: The pulp contains blood vessels, nerves, and connective tissue that are responsible for forming the surrounding dentin and enamel during tooth development. The pulp receives its nourishment supply from vessels that enter the end of the root. Although the pulp is important during development of the tooth, it is not necessary for function of the tooth. The tooth continues to be nourished by the tissues surrounding it even after the pulp is removed.

Question: Why do root canal procedures have such a bad reputation?

Answer: The vast majority of root canal procedures proceed painlessly, both during and after each visit! With modern techniques and anesthetics, people report that having a root canal treatment is about as unremarkable as having a cavity filled. On the other hand, some people present with what we call a hot tooth. A hot tooth is one in which the nerve is alive, but badly inflamed. The tooth is generally already very painful, especially to hot or cold stimuli. These are the ones that require multiple anesthetic injections to get numb.

Question: Is it normal to feel sore after a root canal?

Answer: Yes, it is normal to experience a little soreness after the appointment. This may be due to the injection, the necessity of keeping the mouth open for a long time, or the treatment. The instruments used to remove the pulp from within the tooth can sometimes irritate surrounding tissues causing discomfort for a few days. This is usually minor in most cases. Your temporary filling will be hard enough to bite on within approximately a half-hour, but avoid biting or chewing on the treated tooth if it hurts, especially if there was pain or infection present before the procedure.

Question: What should I do if I am still feeling pain after a root canal?

Answer: Over-the-counter analgesics like acetaminophen, aspirin or ibuprofen usually relieve the discomfort. Other medications can be prescribed as well, but they are rarely required. Should the pain last for more than a few days, or if severe pain or swelling occurs, call your endodontist. Remember, if your tooth hurt before you came in for treatment, it may take a while to heal.

Question: What should I do if I have a swelling (abscess)?

Answer: The first thing you should do if you have an abscess is make an appointment with your dentist to evaluate what the cause of the swelling is and to determine if antibiotics are necessary. For minor swellings caused by gum irritations, hot salt-water rinses may be indicated. Abscesses are usually caused by untreated cavities, cracked teeth, failed root canals or extensive gum disease. There are 3 basic types of abscesses:

- ❖ *Gingival (gum) abscesses* involve only the gum tissue. This is evident as a pus-filled swelling that may have originated from an inflamed periodontal pocket. The dentist will treat this by cleaning out the gum pocket and draining it. Hot rinses and antibiotics may also be needed.
- ❖ A *Traumatic gum abscess* comes from a trauma (such as irritating the area with a toothbrush, or jabbing the gums with something sharp like a crust of bread, chip or bone). Traumatically induced abscesses usually heal on their own with the aid of warm salt water rinses.
- ❖ A *tooth abscess* or *root abscess* involves pus enclosed in the tissues of the jawbone at the tip of an infected tooth. Usually this abscess originates from a bacterial infection that has accumulated within the nerve area of the tooth. In some cases, a tooth abscess may perforate bone and start draining into the surrounding tissues creating local facial swelling. Sometimes the lymph glands in the neck will become swollen and tender in response to the infection. Treatment would be root canal and sometimes antibiotics if the swelling is significant. If you should have any form of swelling, fever or pain, immediately contact your dentist.

Question: What happens if I don't treat a dental abscess?

Answer: A dental abscess is an infection that should be taken very seriously and treated immediately. If the abscess is ignored, not only can it result in a large swelling, fever and intense pain, but it can also have serious consequences, including:

❖ Tooth loss (due to loss of surrounding bone from the infection)

❖ Sinus infection (when the infection from the upper back teeth spread into the neighboring sinuses)

❖ Bacterial Endocarditis (when the bacteria from the abscess spreads to the heart via the blood vessels)

❖ Brain Abscess (when the infection from the abscess reaches the brain through blood vessels)

❖ Osteomyelitis (which is a local or generalized infection of bone and bone marrow, usually caused by the bacteria from the abscess)

❖ Cellulitis (when treatment is delayed, the infection can spread through the tissues and cause facial swelling, fever and can eventually spread to the bone and the soft tissues of the floor of the mouth)

❖ Ludwig's angina (a very serious infection that affects the lower jaw and parts of the face. This infection can grow to block the airways, resulting in suffocation and possibly death)

Question: Couldn't I just have my tooth removed instead of having a root canal?

Answer: You could, but then adjoining teeth may shift and interfere with biting and chewing if you remove the tooth and fail to replace it. You may also consider placing an implant or fill in a missing space with a 'dummy tooth' as part of a fixed or removable bridge. A fixed bridge may require removing adjacent, healthy tooth structure, and may be expensive and require even more dental treatment. If you can save your own tooth with any degree of long-term predictability, then that would always be the first choice.

Question: What happens during root canal treatment?

Answer: An examination, including X-rays, will be performed. A local anesthetic will be given, if necessary. A sheet of latex, called a "rubber dam," will be placed around the tooth to isolate it and keep it clean and dry during treatment. Complete treatment consists of the following five basic steps:

- ❖ Step 1. An opening is made to access the affected nerve tissue (pulp).
- ❖ Step 2. The pulp is removed from within the canals of the roots. Tiny instruments ("files") are used to clean the root canals and shape them to a form that will ensure they will be well sealed. If the root canal is not completed in one visit, then a temporary filling would be placed to seal the opening and protect the tooth between visits.
- ❖ Step 3. The root canals are filled and sealed with a material that prevents bacteria from re-entering. The opening in the crown of the tooth is sealed with a temporary filling. Radiographs (X-rays) are made before, during and after treatment.
- ❖ Step 4. Your dentist will later remove the temporary filling, (ideally within 4 weeks of treatment), and replace it with a more permanent material, to be followed with a permanent restoration or crown.
- ❖ Step 5. The root canal, permanent filling, and/or crown are evaluated for healing at periodic intervals called recall appointments.

Question: How long should my tooth last after having a root canal?

Answer: The answer depends, in part, to how compromised your tooth was to begin with. If there is a lot of good, solid tooth structure to work with, and if your tooth was properly restored with a permanent restoration, then regular brushing and flossing, proper diet and periodic dental check-ups should give your tooth an excellent chance for long term success.

Question: How long can I wait after root canal therapy before I have to get a final restoration?

Answer: When your root canal treatment is complete, a temporary filling is placed. You should then see your general dentist for the permanent crown or restoration. Ideally, the tooth should be permanently restored within a few weeks to prevent the tooth from developing a fracture and to prevent the temporary filling from loosening and leaking, which in turn could cause the root canal treatment to fail, necessitating retreatment.

Question: Does every root canal require a crown (a dental restoration that surrounds the prepared tooth structure?

Answer: Not every root canal requires a crown, however many of them do in order to lend the tooth the proper strength and support. Often times there is not enough tooth structure remaining after a large cavity or fracture to survive without one. Additionally, the tooth can become more brittle after root canal therapy, and would then become more susceptible to fracture, especially if one is a heavy grinder.

Question: What is an apicoectomy?

Answer: Your teeth are held in place by roots that extend into your bone. The tip or end of each root is called the apex. Nerves and blood vessels enter the tooth through the apex. They travel through a canal inside the root, and into the pulp (nerve) chamber. This chamber is inside the crown (the part of the tooth you can see in the mouth). During root canal treatment, the canals are cleaned. Inflamed or infected tissue is removed. An apicoectomy may be needed when an infection develops or won't go away after root canal treatment or retreatment. Root canals are very complex, with many small branches off the main canal. Sometimes, even after root canal treatment, infected debris can remain in these branches. This can possibly prevent healing or cause re-infection later. In an apicoectomy, the root tip, or apex, is removed along with the infected tissue. A filling is then placed to seal the end of the root. An apicoectomy is sometimes called endodontic microsurgery because it is often done using an operating microscope. Most apicoectomies take 30 to 90 minutes. The length will depend on the location of the tooth and the complexity of the root structure.

Procedures on front teeth are generally the shortest. Those on lower molars generally take the longest.

Question: What is an apicoectomy used for?

Answer: If a root canal procedure has been done in the past and it becomes infected again, it's often because of a problem near the apex of the root. In many cases, a second root canal treatment is considered before an apicoectomy. With advances in technology, dentists often can detect other canals that were not adequately treated. In this case, they may be able to clear up the infection by doing a second root canal procedure. This will avoid the need for an apicoectomy. Your dentist can do an apicoectomy to fix the problem so the tooth doesn't need to be extracted. An apicoectomy is done only after a tooth has had at least one root canal procedure and retreatment has not been successful or is not possible. For example, retreatment is often not a good option when a tooth has a crown or is part of a bridge. Retreatment of the root canal would require cutting through the crown or bridge. That might destroy or weaken the crown or bridge. An apicoectomy is often considered in a situation like this. An apicoectomy is not the same as a root resection. In a root resection, an entire root is removed, rather than just the tip.

Question: What does it mean when I get that white pimple-like bump (fistula) on my gum?

Answer: Sometimes after a root canal a pimple develops in the gum area, approximately where the tip of the tooth's root would be. This pimple will often go away and then come back. This is called a fistula. The fistula is a sign that there is an infection and your body is draining it out through the pimple. There is usually no pain in this situation. If you have symptoms, such as pain or a fistula, contact your dentist. He or she will take X-rays and do an exam. If your dentist feels that you may need a root canal or an apicoectomy, then you should set up an appointment for a consultation.

Question: Why do some root canals fail?

Answer: Although only about 5% of root canals fail, there are many possible explanations to explain why this might happen. There may be one or more extra canals that the dentist was unable to locate or fully clean out. This trapped nerve tissue can cause abscesses or ongoing bouts of pain and may lead to failure. A fractured root may cause failure of a root canal. Teeth with dead nerves are always brittle. Fractured roots are generally impossible to repair and this means the loss of the tooth. And in some cases there may be a hypersensitivity to the materials used to fill the canals, although this is a very rare occurrence since the gutta-percha, (a thermoplastic substance from certain trees consisting of a hydrocarbon isometric with rubber) used to fill the canal is quite inert and is generally very well tolerated.

Myth vs. Fact

Myth: Root canal prodeures are painful.

Fact: The vast majority of root canal procedures proceed painlessly, both during and after each visit! With modern techniques and anesthetics, people report that having a root canal treatment is about as unremarkable as having a cavity filled. On the other hand, some people present with what we call a hot tooth. A hot tooth is one in which the nerve is alive, but badly inflamed. The tooth is generally already very painful, especially to hot or cold stimuli. These are the ones that require multiple anesthetic injections to get numb.

9

ORTHODONTICS (BRACES AND INVISALIGN)

Fun Fact...

The first braces were constructed by Pierre Fauchard in 1728 in France. These braces consisted of a flat strip of metal connected to the teeth by pieces of thread.

What it means to get wired...

"The smile, just like life,
requires a bit of push and
pull to set things straight"

Orthodontics was the first dental specialty. It was developed in 1900 out of an interest to create proper occlusion (how teeth come together when they bite). However, orthodontics, in various forms had been attempted before then. In France, 1728, the first set of braces was constructed out of a flat strip of metal connected to the teeth by pieces of thread. We have made many advances since then, from special X-rays and scans to better diagnose, to surgical procedures to better correct poor growth patterns of the jaw. Braces themselves are less of an eyesore, and clear orthodontic retainers (i.e. Invisalign) can often be used to correct misaligned teeth.

Crooked teeth and a poor bite are a regular finding that, aside from not being as esthetic, can contribute to tooth decay and gum disease, (being harder to clean and maintain), and can place an additional stress on the chewing muscles, resulting in headaches, TMJ problems and neck, shoulder and back pain. When treatment is started early in childhood, orthodontic treatment can help to allow for proper jaw growth and eruption of the permanent teeth. Orthodontics is now considered a predictable and necessary treatment to create and restore beauty and health to the mouth.

Orthodontics

Question: What is an orthodontist?

Answer: An orthodontist not only specializes in straightening teeth, but also specializes in the diagnosis, prevention and treatment of dental and facial irregularities. Orthodontists receive two or more years of education beyond their four years in dental school in an ADA-approved orthodontic training program. Their care involves the use of corrective appliances, such as braces, in order to: straighten teeth, correct bite irregularities, close unsightly gaps, and bring teeth and lips into proper alignment.

Question: What is orthodontics?

Answer: Orthodontics is the branch of dentistry that corrects teeth and jaws that are positioned improperly. Crooked teeth and teeth that do not fit together correctly are harder to keep clean are at risk of being lost early due to tooth decay and periodontal disease, and cause extra stress on the chewing muscles that can lead to headaches, TMJ syndrome and neck, shoulder and back pain. Teeth that are crooked or not in the right place can also detract from one's appearance. The benefits of orthodontic treatment include a healthier mouth, a more pleasing appearance, and teeth that are more likely to last a lifetime. Orthodontics can also be used to help with procedures in other areas of dentistry, such as cosmetic dentistry or implant dentistry, where space may need to be added or eliminated. In young children, orthodontic treatment helps to guide proper jaw growth and permanent tooth eruption.

Question: How do I know if I am a candidate for braces or some other form of orthodontics?

Answer: Your dentist or orthodontist can determine whether you can benefit from orthodontic treatment. They base their decision on diagnostic tools that include a full medical and dental health history, a clinical exam, plaster models of your teeth, and special X-rays and photographs.

If you have any of the following, you may be a candidate for orthodontic treatment:

- ❖ **Overbite**, sometimes called "buck teeth" — where the upper front teeth lie too far forward (stick out) over the lower teeth
- ❖ **Underbite** — a "bulldog" appearance where the lower teeth are too far forward or the upper teeth too far back
- ❖ **Crossbite** — when the upper teeth do not slightly overlap the lower teeth when biting together normally as they should, but rather the lower teeth are overlapping the uppers
- ❖ **Open bite** — space between the biting surfaces of the front and/or side teeth when the back teeth bite together
- ❖ **Misplaced midline**— when the center of your upper front teeth does not line up with the center of your lower front teeth
- ❖ **Spacing** — gaps, or spaces, between the teeth that occur naturally, or as a result of missing teeth
- ❖ **Crowding** — when there are too many teeth for the upper and lower jaws to accommodate

Question: How does orthodontic treatment work?

Answer: Many different types of appliances, both fixed and removable, are used to help move teeth, retrain muscles and affect the growth of the jaws. These appliances work by placing gentle pressure on the teeth and jaws.

Fixed appliances include:

❖ **Braces** — the most common fixed appliances, braces consist of bands, wires and/or brackets. Bands are fixed around the teeth or tooth and used as anchors for the appliance, while brackets are most often bonded to the front of the tooth. Arch wires are passed through the brackets and attached to the bands. Tightening the arch wire puts tension on the teeth, gradually moving them to their proper position. Braces are usually adjusted monthly to bring about the desired results, which may be achieved within a few months to a few years. Today's braces are smaller, lighter and show far less metal than in the past. They come in bright colors for kids as well as clear styles preferred by many adults.

❖ **Special fixed appliances** — used to control thumb sucking or tongue thrusting, these appliances are attached to the teeth by bands. Because they are very uncomfortable during meals, they should be used only as a last resort.

❖ **Fixed space maintainers** — if a baby tooth is lost prematurely, a space maintainer is used to keep the space open until the permanent tooth erupts. A band is attached to the tooth next to the empty space, and a wire is extended to the tooth on the other side of the space.

Removable appliances include:

❖ **Aligners (i.e. Invisalign)** — an alternative to traditional braces for adults, serial aligners are being used by an increasing number of orthodontists to move teeth in the same way that fixed appliances work, only without metal wires and brackets. Aligners are virtually invisible and are removed for eating, brushing and flossing.

❖ **Removable space maintainers** — these devices serve the same function as fixed space maintainers. They're made with an acrylic base that fits over the jaw, and have plastic or wire branches between specific teeth to keep the space between them open.

❖ **Jaw repositioning appliances** — also called splints, these devices are worn on either on the top or lower jaw, and help train the jaw to close in a more favorable position. They may be used for temporomandibular joint disorders (TMJ).

❖ **Lip and cheek bumpers** — these are designed to keep the lips or cheeks away from the teeth. Lip and cheek muscles can exert pressure on the teeth, and these bumpers help relieve that pressure.

❖ **Palatal expander** — a device used to widen the arch of the upper jaw. It is a plastic plate that fits over the roof of the mouth. Outward pressure applied to the plate by screws force the joints in the bones of the palate to open lengthwise, widening the palatal area.

❖ **Removable retainers** — worn on the roof of the mouth, these devices prevent shifting of the teeth to their previous position. They can also be modified and used to prevent thumb sucking.

❖ **Headgear** — with this device, a strap is placed around the back of the head and attached to a metal wire in front, or face bow. Headgear slows the growth of the upper jaw, and holds the back teeth where they are while the front teeth are pulled back.

Question: Does having orthodontics early on mean less treatment later?

Answer: Orthodontic treatment in young children is known as interceptive orthodontics, in which intervention begins before the child starts first grade. At this age, tooth development and jaw growth have not been completed, so certain conditions, like crowding, are easier to address. Before permanent teeth have come in, it may be possible to help teeth to erupt (emerge through the gums) into the proper positions. It's common, for example, for the dental arch to be too small to accommodate all of the teeth. A few decades ago, the solution for crowding was to extract some of the adult teeth and use fixed braces to position the teeth properly. Early intervention takes advantage of the fact that a child's jaw is still growing. For example, a device called a palatal expander may be used to expand the child's upper arch. Once the arch is the proper size, there's a better chance that the adult teeth will emerge naturally where they should. If all teeth have erupted and there is still a great deal of crowding, some permanent teeth may have to be extracted to align the teeth properly. Children who receive interceptive orthodontics may still need braces or other orthodontic appliances later. However, this early treatment may shorten and simplify future treatment and may eliminate the need for more drastic measures such as the need to extract permanent teeth in the future.

Question: Are braces hard to get used to?

Answer: Braces today tend to be less uncomfortable and less visible than they used to be, but they still take some getting used to. Food can get caught in the wires, flossing and brushing can take more time, and after the monthly adjustments sometimes the teeth are a little sore. Tooth discomfort can be controlled by taking an analgesic such Advil, Motrin, Tylenol and others. The use of lighter and more flexible wires has greatly lessened the amount of soreness or discomfort during treatment. Because treatment has become more socially acceptable, social embarrassment may be less of a concern.

Question: Does it still pay to have orthodontics as an adult?

Answer: Whether or not one should seek orthodontic care at an older age is an individual decision. Many people live with crowding, overbites or other types of alignment problems without the motivation to seek orthodontic treatment. However, many people feel more comfortable and self-confident with properly aligned, attractive teeth. Unlike strictly cosmetic procedures, orthodontic care can also benefit your long-term dental health. Straight, properly aligned teeth are easier to maintain with proper oral hygiene, such as flossing and brushing. This can help reduce the risk of cavities as well as gum disease, which occurs more readily as it becomes increasingly more difficult to clean around crowded and rotated teeth. In addition, people with bad bites may chew less efficiently. In severe cases, (particularly when the jaws are not aligned correctly), this can result in nutritional deficiencies. Correcting bite irregularities can make it easier to chew and digest foods.

Improperly coordinated upper and lower front teeth also can create speech difficulties, which can be corrected through orthodontic treatment.

Finally, orthodontic treatment can help to prevent premature wear of back tooth surfaces. As you bite down, your teeth withstand a tremendous amount of force. If your front teeth don't meet properly, it can cause your back teeth to wear more.

Question: What are the different ways to close a gap without using braces?

Answer: While braces are a fairly common and predictable way to close a gap between teeth, it is sometimes necessary to explore other options that would be better suited for one's needs. Among these options are porcelain veneers (thin pieces of porcelain that are made in a dental lab and then bonded into place to create the illusion of a more perfect smile), and bonding (using tooth-colored, composite resin to fill in the spaces between teeth). Both techniques can fix the gaps in one's smile fairly quickly (within 2 weeks for the veneers, and within an hour or two for the bonding). Bonding will most likely be the more cost-effective way of achieving your goals, but may require periodic maintenance and may not be as natural looking as the porcelain veneer option.

Question: What is *Invisalign®*?

Answer: Invisalign® straightens your teeth with a series of clear, virtually invisible custom-molded aligners that are made from digital scans or impressions taken by your dentist or orthodontist. Unlike braces, *Invisalign®* aligners have no metal bands or wires to irritate your mouth. Since *Invisalign®* is removable, you can take the clear aligner out for meals, brushing and special events, although you will need to wear your trays for at least 21 hours a day for it to be effective. *Invisalign®* also allows you to view your own virtual treatment plan before you start so you can see how straight your teeth will look once your treatment is complete.

Question: What should I expect when I get braces?

Answer: Braces work by applying continuous pressure to move teeth in a specific direction. Braces are worn for an average of one to three years. As treatment progresses, teeth change position, and the braces must be adjusted. When applying braces, the orthodontist will attach tiny brackets to your teeth with special dental bonding agents. He or she will then place wires called arch wires through the brackets. The arch wires, which usually are made of a variety of alloys, act as tracks to create the "path of movement" that guides the teeth. Wires made of clear or tooth-colored materials are less visible than stainless steel wires but are more expensive. Tiny elastic bands hold the arch wires to the brackets, and patients can choose from a multitude of colors at each visit. Expect to be uncomfortable for the first few days after getting braces. Your teeth may be sore, and the wires, brackets and bands may irritate your tongue, cheeks or lips. Most of the discomfort disappears within a week or two, although you may experience moderate pain when wires are changed or adjusted. Taking ibuprofen (Motrin, Advil) or other over-the-counter painkillers can help to ease any discomfort.

Question: Do I have to wear metal braces, or are there other options?

Answer: You can choose between braces made of metal, ceramic or plastic. However, orthodontic treatment usually is done using stainless steel brackets. Ceramic or plastic brackets often are chosen for cosmetic reasons, but plastic brackets may stain and discolor by the end of treatment. Bands made of plastic or ceramic also have more friction between the wire and brackets, which can increase treatment time. Other options for adults include *Invisalign*®, which is a series of clear retainers designed to move teeth into proper alignment, but may have certain limitations when it comes to more advanced tooth movements.

Question: Why do I need to wear a retainer?

Answer: A retainer's purpose is to maintain tooth positions after corrective orthodontic treatment. Once your bite has been corrected, bone and gums need additional time to stabilize around the teeth. The recommended length of time for wearing a retainer varies from orthodontist to orthodontist. Most children and teenagers wear retainers until they reach their early to mid-20's, but your orthodontist's recommendation should be followed strictly because he or she knows your treatment best. You can choose from a removable retainer or a fixed wire retainer that gets bonded to the inside surface of your teeth to prevent relapse and movement.

Question: What happens if you don't wear your retainer all the time?

Answer: If you don't wear your retainer you will run the risk of your teeth shifting back to their original position. The ligaments around the teeth have memory, and the more rotated your teeth were before, the more likely they will drift back without the proper retention. It is most important to wear your retainer for the first 6 months following orthodontic treatment, so that the bone around the teeth will have a better chance to fully fill in the areas from around where the tooth was moved. After this time it is recommended to continue wearing your retainers, unless you are told otherwise by your dentist or orthodontist. At the very least, you should try in your retainer every few days to make sure that it isn't fitting too tight, signaling some drifting may be taking place. A permanent metal wire splinted to the inside of your front teeth can eliminate the need for the removable retainer, and help to maintain your straightened teeth if you are prone to being non-compliant.

Question: How should I take care of my retainer?

Answer: Most retainers are removable, meaning that you take them out when eating, brushing and flossing. For this reason, they are easy to misplace. Many people wrap their retainers in a napkin when eating, then forget about them afterwards and have to spend hundreds of dollars on a new retainer. A good solution is to always carry your retainer case with you and to use it whenever you're not wearing your retainer. For added protection, never leave the case on a table or a bench — always put it immediately in your backpack, purse or pocket.

Your dentist can give you information on how to clean and care for your specific type of retainer. Regardless of the type, you need to make sure you don't sit on, step on or otherwise damage this delicate and expensive piece of equipment.

Question: What should I do to fix my braces if a bracket or band comes lose or a wire breaks or sticks out?

Answer: Braces, bands or the wires that are affixed to each tooth occasionally will break or fall off completely, but usually what happens is that one of the parts will loosen, which may cause minor discomfort. Here are a few problems that can occur:

❖ **Loose bracket** — Brackets are the metal or ceramic pieces that are bonded (glued) to the teeth. If the bond weakens or breaks, which can happen after you chew something hard or sticky, the bracket can dislodge and may poke at the gum tissue or other soft tissues in the mouth, such as your tongue or cheek. You can temporarily reattach loose brackets with a small piece of orthodontic wax, or place wax over the bracket to provide a cushion so it doesn't poke you. This should provide some comfort until you can see your orthodontist.

❖ **Loose band** — Orthodontic bands are the metal rings cemented with dental bonding agents or cement around back teeth. If an orthodontic band becomes loose, call for an appointment to have it re-cemented or replaced. If the band comes off the tooth or the wire completely, do not replace it yourself. Save the band and call to schedule an appointment for repair.

❖ **Protruding or broken wire** — This is a common problem. If a wire sticks out of the bracket or band or breaks, it may poke or damage your cheek, tongue or gum. The easiest solution is to use the eraser end of a pencil to push the wire into a less bothersome position. If you can't bend it out of the way, put a small piece of orthodontic wax over the end that is sticking out. You should not cut the orthodontic wire yourself. A cut wire can be accidentally swallowed or inhaled into your lungs. If the damaged wire has caused a painful sore, rinse your mouth with warm salt water or an antiseptic rinse. This will keep the area clean and help reduce the discomfort. You can also apply an over-the-counter dental anesthetic (pain reliever), which will temporarily numb the area. If you are not feeling better, or the wire is still irritating you, contact your orthodontist ASAP so they can adjust the wire.

❖ **Loose spacer** — Spacers or separators are rubber circular pieces that are put between your teeth. They are left in place for a brief period of time, usually for several days. They open a small space between your teeth so that the orthodontic band will slip into place easily. Sometimes, they can slip out of position or fall out entirely. If this happens you should make an appointment with your orthodontist to have them replaced.

Question: Do I need to spend more time caring for my teeth when wearing braces?

Answer: Yes, a lot of extra care is needed during orthodontics. The brackets and wires have many nooks and crannies that can trap food and plaque. This means your risk of tooth decay and gum problems may be higher while you are wearing braces. You need to pay special attention to cleaning your teeth everyday and to your diet (try to avoid acidic foods and beverages like soda). Permanent damage to tooth enamel can occur if the teeth and brackets are not kept clean, such as unsightly white spots due to the enamel becoming demineralized. Most of us are well aware that sugary foods and drinks can lead to tooth decay, but starchy foods, such as potato chips, and foods like nuts and raisins can also stick to teeth for long periods of time and cause tooth decay. Avoid hard foods such as nuts and hard cookies. There are foods that can loosen, break or bend wires and bands when you are wearing braces. Foods such as apples and carrots should be chopped into small pieces before eating to reduce the stress on your braces. Avoid sticky foods such as caramels, toffees, or fruit bars. No chewing gum! No chewing ice! Drink plenty of water, and use fluoride toothpastes and rinses as recommended by your orthodontist. Additionally, try to avoid giving in to bad habits such as nail biting, unnatural tongue thrusting, pencil chewing and picking at your wires, which can also break your braces. Consider using special electric brush tips or orthodontic brushes, along with a waterpik and floss threaders to clean more efficiently. While you are having orthodontic treatment, you need to continue to have regular check-ups with your dental professional to ensure that little problems don't become big ones.

Question: Is there any way to prevent the need for braces?

Answer: If your mouth is destined to become crowded, or to develop large gaps or rotations, then braces are most likely in your future. However, there are ways to limit the duration of the treatment, or make it less involved. If you are seen early enough to do some interceptive orthodontics to correct conditions such as a constricted palate or cross bite, the treatment when you are older will be less complicated and much less time consuming. Additionally, wearing your retainers will prevent the need for braces again in the future. Some individuals, who are candidates, may also choose to wear *Invisalign*® trays (clear, plastic orthodontic trays) to straighten teeth instead of opting for the bracket, band and wire option of traditional braces.

Myth vs. Fact

Myth: If the appearance of my teeth doesn't bother me, there is no point in getting braces or *Invisalign* ®.

Fact: Whether or not one should seek orthodontic care at an older age is an individual decision. Many people live with crowding, overbites or other types of alignment problems without the motivation to seek orthodontic treatment. However, many people feel more comfortable and self-confident with properly aligned, attractive teeth. Unlike strictly cosmetic procedures, orthodontic care can also benefit your long-term dental health. Straight, properly aligned teeth are easier to maintain with proper oral hygiene, such as flossing and brushing. This can help reduce the risk of cavities as well as gum disease, which occurs more readily as it becomes increasingly more difficult to clean around crowded and rotated teeth. In addition, people with bad bites may chew less efficiently. In severe cases, (particularly when the jaws are not aligned correctly), this can result in nutritional deficiencies. Correcting bite irregularities can make it easier to chew and digest foods. Improperly coordinated upper and lower front teeth also can create speech difficulties, which can be corrected through orthodontic treatment.

Finally, orthodontic treatment can help to prevent premature wear of back tooth surfaces. As you bite down, your teeth withstand a tremendous amount of force. If your front teeth don't meet properly, it can cause your back teeth to wear more.

10

Pediatrics (Children's Dental Care)

Fun Fact...

Children smile about 400 times a day,
while grown-ups average just 15.

If you have kids, read this...

"Little teeth can still cause big problems"

The dental profession continues to reinforce its commitment to delivering the best care possible to children while constantly re-examining the way in which this care is being conducted. Over the years new advances have enhanced the quality of care delivered, from the introduction of fluoride in our water supply to the advances in orthodontic and preventative treatments. With new technology and research come new philosophies and mindsets, all of which contribute to creating healthy, beautiful smiles that will last a lifetime. More and more, dental healthcare providers are taking time to educate their patients on ways to maintain preventative dental habits, with a special emphasis on preventing tooth decay. Proper care will prevent premature loss of children's teeth, which can affect their speech development, social relationships, psychology and self-image. Children's first dental experiences can often affect their life-long attitudes towards dental care. This chapter explores all aspects of children's dental care, from tooth development and home care techniques, to fluoride and preventative care.

Pediatric Dental Care
(Children's Dental Care)

Question: What is a pediatric dentist?

Answer: A pediatric dentist (formerly pedodontist) specializes in the oral health care needs of young people, including infants, children and adolescents. Pediatric dentists have completed an additional 2-3 years of study and hands-on training after dental school, to prepare them to aid in the unique dental needs of their younger population. If your general dentist feels your child needs unusual procedures or might be difficult to treat, you may be referred to a pediatric dentist.

Question: When will my infant's primary teeth (aka deciduous or baby teeth) grow in, and how do you care for them?

Answer: A baby's first tooth will usually erupt into the mouth by around six months of age. Some infants will be early, and some may be a few months later. If your baby still has not displayed their first tooth by the time they are 1 year old, then you can bring your child to the dentist for an exam. *From day one* you should be cleaning your baby's gums, and tongue with a washcloth, rubber finger brush, or cloth finger tender (even though no teeth are present). Clean the gums at least twice each day -- after breakfast and after the last feeding of the day. Even better -- clean your baby's gums and tongue after every feeding to keep the breath fresh and to get them accustomed to this routine. Once the first tooth erupts, you should be cleaning these teeth, trading in your cloth wipe for an appropriate sized, soft toothbrush. In order to see the teeth more clearly when brushing, you may choose to have your child lay their head on your lap, or lay them down on a bed. Remember to only use toothpaste that does NOT contain fluoride at this time.

Baby (Primary) Teeth Development Chart		
Upper Teeth	When tooth emerges	When tooth falls out
Central incisor	8 to 12 months	6 to 7 years
Lateral incisor	9 to 13 months	7 to 8 years

Canine (cuspid)	16 to 22 months	10 to 12 years
First molar	13 to 19 months	9 to 11 years
Second molar	25 to 33 months	10 to 12 years
Lower Teeth		
Second molar	23 to 31 months	10 to 12 years
First molar	14 to 18 months	9 to 11 years
Canine (cuspid)	17 to 23 months	9 to 12 years
Lateral incisor	10 to 16 months	7 to 8 years
Central incisor	6 to 10 months	6 to 7 years

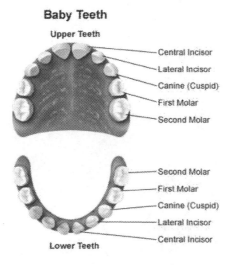

Baby Teeth

Question: What can be done to prevent baby teeth from developing cavities?

Answer: Parents and caregivers should realize that a baby's teeth are susceptible to developing cavities from the moment they appear in the mouth. As a result, oral care should begin soon after the baby is born, and their gums should be cleaned with a clean, damp cloth or wet gauze pad after each feeding. As early as 4 months or as late as 12 months of age, the upper and lower front teeth first begin to appear. You may begin brushing your child's teeth the moment these teeth emerge. Never let your baby or toddler fall asleep with a bottle, unless it contains only pure water. Make sure the bottle is rinsed out well before being filled. A bottle containing milk, formula, fruit juices, etc., is likely to cause decay. A pacifier coated with a sugary substance is also likely to cause cavities. This condition is referred to as Baby Bottle Tooth Decay, or Nursing-Bottle Syndrome. The teeth most likely to be affected are the upper front teeth, but other teeth can become damaged as well.

Question: Why are baby teeth important?

Answer: Baby teeth hold the space for the permanent teeth, which begin coming in at about 6 years of age. Your baby's teeth, gums and tongue are not only very important for eating, but aid in the growth pattern of your child's jaws and adult teeth. Note that baby teeth are also a key component in the ability to learn and perfect speech. Of course, a full complement of baby teeth will contribute to having a good self-image as your child grows older.

Question: When will my child's adult teeth grow in, and how do I care for them?

Answer: Spaces for the permanent teeth begin to appear at the age of 4 as the jaw, supporting bone structure and facial bones begin to grow. The first baby teeth to be lost are the two lower front teeth. These come out between 6-7 years of age and are very soon replaced with the two lower adult front teeth. At the same time, the 6 year molars are starting to grow in. From 6-12, it is typical for your child to have a combination of both baby teeth and permanent teeth in their mouth. Below is a chart showing when to expect the emergence of all the adult teeth.

Adult (Permanent) Teeth Development Chart	
Upper Teeth	**When tooth emerges**
Central incisor	7 to 8 years
Lateral incisor	8 to 9 years
Canine (cuspid)	11 to 12 years
First premolar (first bicuspid)	10 to 11 years
Second premolar (second bicuspid)	10 to 12 years
First molar	6 to 7 years
Second molar	12 to 13 years

Third molar (wisdom teeth)	17 to 21 years
Lower Teeth	
Third molar (wisdom tooth)	17 to 21 years
Second molar	11 to 13 years
First molar	6 to 7 years
Second premolar (second bicuspid)	11 to 12 years
First premolar (first bicuspid)	10 to 12 years
Canine (cuspid)	9 to 10 years
Lateral incisor	7 to 8 years
Central incisor	6 to 7 years

Question: What can I do if I have difficulty cleaning my baby's mouth?

Answer: If your baby does not want to open their mouth, place your finger near their mouth, and they will slowly open as they think that you are trying to feed them. Even if your baby tries to bite down on your finger, be patient, keep trying, and they will soon open up again. Reach inside along the cheek until you get between the upper and lower gums, and your baby will then open more to allow you to wipe the gums in the very back. If it is the case that one or more ulcers are found in your baby's mouth, just clean around the ulcers until they are healed (usually within one week). Get your child accustomed to cleaning his/her mouth regularly and going to bed with a clean mouth.

Question: Is it alright to let my baby sleep with a pacifier, sippy cup or bottle?

Answer: If your child uses a pacifier, do not dip it in honey or anything that has sugar, as this can cause cavities. Do not put your child to bed with a bottle or sippy cup that contains milk, formula, fruit juices or soda, since these contain sugary substances that can cause cavities too. Plain water is the only acceptable fluid to give your child when they are going to nap or sleep for the night.

Question: How do I control my child's drooling and teething pain?

Answer: Babies can be very easily agitated by the teething process. Parents should try to distract their children with activities, and allow their child to chew on a clean, chilled, liquid-filled teething ring to relieve the discomfort and irritation. Drooling during this time is normal and expected. Just wipe your child's mouth often to keep them clean and dry. Swollen gums are normal at this time; however if the gum turns blue or red, then bring your child to the dentist to evaluate. Additionally, teething should not cause fever. Since your baby is picking up anything and everything that has germs on it, and putting it in their mouth to chew on, it is possible that their fever is due to this spreading of illness, in which case parents should bring their child to their pediatrician.

Question: I heard that sometimes a baby could be born with one or more teeth (natal teeth), if that happens what should I do?

Answer: Occasionally a baby may be born with teeth (natal teeth) or erupt through the gums within the first month of life (neonatal teeth). Their occurrence is about 1 in 30,000 and usually just the lower front baby teeth; posterior tooth eruption is extremely rare. These teeth are usually the normal baby lower front teeth erupting early. Due to this early eruption, the tooth will not be fully developed. If this should occur, leave them alone, unless they are very loose or causing traumatic ulcers, or causing any discomfort to the baby or mother during breast-feeding, in which case you would have them removed. This is a non-traumatic procedure and painless to the infant. Because natal and neonatal teeth are usually normal baby teeth, a new baby tooth will not replace them once they are lost. The space is usually left alone until the adult teeth eventually grow into that area. Teeth that are stable after 4 months have a good prognosis, although they may be discolored and not as esthetically pleasing as the other teeth.

Question: When should I first take my child to the dentist?

Answer: Parents should take their children to the dentist for their first check-up by the age of 2, unless your doctor recommends an earlier exam. Subsequently, they should go for regular check-ups every 6 months, so your child's dentist can monitor their oral hygiene, diet and growth patterns. It is best if your child's first experience occurs at a time before invasive dental work becomes necessary. A ride on the dental chair, magic tricks with "Mr. Thirsty" (dental suction tool) and visiting the toy chest should make your child's visit pleasurable and non-threatening. The first visit should also include the counting of teeth while your child looks at what is happening in a hand-held mirror. Remember, early dental check-up makes it easier to build a good rapport with your child to establish a foundation of trust and comfort for future visits.

Question: How should I prepare my child for their dental visits?

Answer: Tell your child that the dentist is there to help take care of his/her teeth. Read your child a fun children's book about going to the dentist. Describe to your child the surroundings of a dental office and you can role play the job of a dentist. It may help to tell your child the date for the dental visit, in advance, so that they can prepare for the visit and hopefully look forward to it. Remember, NEVER use the dentist as a threat for not taking care of their teeth, this will just instill a fear in them that will last well into the future. Speak positively about dental visits, and make it something to look forward to. It is important to establish a positive relationship between your child and the dentist by starling early and continuing to see the dentist for regular check-ups. And don't forget to share this valuable knowledge with anyone else who may be helping to care for your child.

Question: When does my child need fluoride, and what is the right amount?

Answer: Fluoride is a mineral that helps to prevent tooth decay by strengthening the tooth's enamel and making it more resistant to acids and harmful bacteria. Most municipal water supplies are fortified with fluoride (check with your local water authority to find out about yours). Some bottled water companies will fortify some of their water products with fluoride, so be sure to check the labels. If the fluoride content of your water supply has less than 0.3 parts per million, ask your child's doctor whether you should give your child a fluoride supplement (the amount recommended for children from 6 months-3yrs old is 0.25 milligrams per day). Your doctor can prescribe fluoride in the form of drops that you can add to your baby's bottle or food once per day, or they can be prescribed as part of your child's vitamin. The American Academy of Pediatrics doesn't recommend fluoride supplements for babies under 6 months old. Your child will not get any fluoride from breast milk. If you live in an area with fluoridated water, your child will get fluoride from the water you use to make the formula. A little fluoride is good for your baby's teeth, but too much of it can lead to a condition called fluorosis, which can cause white spots on your child's adult teeth. It is recommended to wait until your child is old enough to spit out before giving your child fluoridated toothpaste, and even then you should let them use only a tiny (pea-sized) amount each time. This is because young children tend to swallow their toothpaste rather than spit it out and swallowing too much toothpaste over time can lead to fluorosis, or become toxic in large quantities.

Age	Fluoride Ion Level in Drinking Water (ppm)*		
	<0.3 ppm	0.3-0.6 ppm	>0.6 ppm
Birth-6 months	None	None	None
6 months-3 years	0.25 mg/day**	None	None
3-6 years	0.50 mg/day	0.25 mg/day	None
6-16 years	1.0 mg/day	0.50 mg/day	None
* 1.0 ppm = 1 mg/liter			
** 2.2 mg sodium fluoride contains 1 mg fluoride ion.			

Question: Can water filters reduce the benefits a fluoridated water system would otherwise offer to my children's teeth?

Answer: Yes, some types of water treatment systems that are installed in one's home can decrease the fluoride levels, thus potentially reducing the cavity-preventing effects of a water supply that has been optimally fluoridated. It has been documented that the reverse osmosis systems and distillation units remove significant amounts of fluoride. However, studies have also shown that water softeners do not cause a significant loss in fluoride levels. The concentration of fluoride found in your water will depend on the type and quality of the water filter you purchased, the current status of the filter and its age. For questions about the level of fluoride in your water supply or to arrange to have your filtered water tested, contact your local and state public health departments. Your dentist should also be contacted to determine if your children are candidates for fluoride supplementation, as it is available by prescription only. Those individuals who drink bottled water as their primary source of water may also be depriving themselves of the benefits of fluoride, as many brands fall short of the optimum levels of 0.7 ppm.

Question: Is it better to use a manual toothbrush or an electric toothbrush for my child's teeth?

Answer: An electric brush has a few advantages over a manual brush. First it generates more brush strokes per second; making it more effective for the amount of time it is being used. Keep in mind that while it is recommended to brush for 2 minutes, the average person only brushes for 30 seconds. With an electric brush it is easier to clean behind the back teeth. Many of these electric brushes have certain extra bells and whistles such as a digital timer so you know when 2 minutes are up, and an indicator light to show if you are pressing too hard. There is usually less trauma to the gums and teeth when brushing with an electric brush since many overzealous manual toothbrush users bang into their gums with the wrong technique, or scrub too hard. A manual toothbrush can be very effective with the right technique, and conversely, an electric toothbrush can be virtually useless with the wrong technique. If using a manual brush, use small, vibratory strokes on a 45-degree angle so that the bristles get in the pockets between the teeth and gums. Avoid the up and down or circular motion, as that can just traumatize the gums. If you are using an electric brush, try to spend at least 2 full seconds on each tooth surface, (inside, outside and top), making sure to angle the brush between the teeth and having the bristles go between the tooth and the gums. Spin brushes are just a watered down version of an electric brush that may attract the attention of your child with its various themed versions. Whether you use a manual brush or an electric one, make sure you always change your brush or brush head every three months, or sooner, if you just had a cold so you don't reinfect yourself.

Question: At what age should a child brush their teeth on their own?

Answer: This will depend on the child. While it is great to build up a child's self-confidence and independence, children do not usually develop the full coordination and understanding of what they are trying to accomplish until the age of 6 or 7. Even though they may want to do this all by themselves, it is recommended that the parent or guardian supervise, check, and when necessary, do additional brushing for their child at least up until the age of 10. Your toddler can have their toothbrush available for "pretend or play" tooth-brushing along with you. Cavities prevented during this time will save a lot of time, money and trauma in the future.

Question: How often should I brush my child's teeth, and at what times of the day?

Answer: It is recommended that everyone brush at least twice each day with a soft-bristled brush or electric brush. The first time should be in the morning, after breakfast, so your child's teeth are clean before leaving for school. It defeats the purpose of brushing if you give your child their sugary vitamin after they brush, or give them their breakfast to nibble on the bus, because these substances will stay lodged in the top grooves of their molars and in between their teeth for hours to come, contributing to the formation of cavities. The most important time to brush is right before you go to sleep at night so that nothing is left on or in between your teeth when you are sleeping. The reason is that when you are awake, your saliva helps to bathe and rinse your teeth, but while asleep, you do not salivate that much, and your teeth are more susceptible to developing cavities from the debris left on them. Additionally, if you have the chance to brush after other meals or snacks, it would be advisable. And don't forget to brush their teeth after they are given medicine, as the acids contained in medicines may break down the tooth enamel.

Question: When should my child start flossing?

Answer: Parent-assisted dental flossing is recommended as soon as the teeth erupt next to each other. Independent flossing is recommended once children develop the dexterity to be able to do it on their own (often by 6 or 7 years of age).

Question: Which foods are bad for my child's teeth?

Answer: Any food or snack that can become trapped within the pits and grooves of your child's teeth or between their teeth can become harmful if not cleaned properly. Chewy candy (i.e. taffies, caramels, jellybeans, and licorice) are among the biggest cavity culprits. However, you may be surprised to know that nuts, raisins and dried fruits can also cause a lot of damage, since they too get readily stuck in and around the teeth. The complex carbohydrates such as pretzels and potato chips get broken down into the same sugars that are found in cakes and cookies. Any food debris left on the tooth creates an acid attack in the mouth which breaks it down. The less likely the food is to dissolve or rinse away, the longer the acid attacks will be. Chocolate, which is full of sugar, is actually not as bad for your teeth as dried fruit and nuts, because chocolate dissolves quickly. However, you can prolong any acid attack by eating or drinking things slowly over a longer period of time.

Question: What are dental sealants and what do they do?

Answer: Aside from the introduction of fluoride, dental sealants have become one of the biggest breakthroughs in terms of dental prevention. They are used to protect teeth from decay and are appropriate as soon as a posterior tooth erupts. The chewing surfaces of these back teeth have many pits and grooves that can trap food debris and cause cavities. Children and adults alike can benefit from dental sealants, which are a plastic resin that flows into the cleaned out grooves of the tooth, and hardened to make a more shallow, ice-skating like surface for which the food debris can be more readily brushed away. Sealants should be checked at your regular dental visits and redone periodically if wear or breakdown is evident.

Question: What do I do if my toddler won't let me brush his/her teeth?

Answer: There are a few techniques that you can pull out of your arsenal. The first is to have several different fun toothbrushes to choose from. When you go to brush their teeth with one of them, they will reach out and grab it from you. Then you pick up another brush and try to brush their teeth with that one knowing that they will now grab that brush from you with their other free hand. Now that both of their hands are occupied, you can go in with a third brush, preferably an electric one so you can get more accomplished in less time. Another technique is to say all the things you might see in there, recalling their meals and snacks that day as you brush (i.e. "I see a little pretzel there, let me get that away…. oh look a piece of chicken, let me get that piece of cookie out…," etc.). You can try brushing to music, while they are watching a show, or while doing anything that is fun and creative. If all else fails, then try the two-person technique where one person holds the legs down and the other straddles the head while pinning their straight arms along the side of their head. They will cry and scream, which is good because their mouths will now be wide open. Within several times of doing this they will start to realize that it is just easier to allow you to brush their teeth without resistance, and they won't remember this experience anyway.

Question: My baby has white patches inside the mouth. What causes this?

Answer: It most likely could be caused by a common and harmless yeast infection known as thrush. Thrush (also known as Oral Candidiasis) looks like cottage cheese on the sides, roof, and sometimes the tongue of a baby's mouth. Usually you will find it in babies 2 months and younger, but it can appear in older babies as well. What happens is that after your baby is born, antibiotics taken by you, (if you're breastfeeding), or your baby, can trigger a case of thrush. These antibiotics kill off the "good" bacteria that can prevent a yeast imbalance. Often moms and babies pass the infection back and forth: Your baby can pass thrush on to you if you're breastfeeding, resulting in a painful yeast infection on your nipples that would require a doctor's treatment. And you can trigger a case of thrush in your baby if you're breastfeeding and you develop a yeast infection on your nipples from taking antibiotics.

Question: What is primary herpetic gingivostomatitis?

Answer: It is caused by an initial infection with the Herpes simplex virus Type I and is characterized by painful, red, and swollen gums. Multiple little vesicles first present around the border of the mouth. The vesicles soon rupture into large, painful ulcers. Symptoms include: fever, malaise and swollen lymph nodes, followed by the appearance of the vesicles that progress into ulcers. Most common age is 6 months to 6 years. This condition is contagious, until the lesions spontaneously heal within 1-2 weeks. Treatment includes: rest, fever and pain medications (no antibiotics unless there is a secondary infection present). Certain mouth rinses may help with oral discomfort. Petroleum jelly or Orabase gel may be used as a protective barrier. Dehydration may be a concern, especially in a younger patient.

Question: Does it really matter if my child has a cavity in their baby tooth; they will lose it soon anyway?

Answer: Yes, it does matter. Baby molars enter the mouth around the age of 2 years old. If a cavity develops early on, that cavity is only going to keep growing down deeper towards the nerve. Since these baby molars aren't lost until the age of 10-12 years of age, there is plenty of time for unnecessary, preventable damage to occur. As the cavity grows, the child may wind up needing a baby root canal or an extraction if an infection develops or if there not enough good tooth structure to utilize for a restoration. These baby teeth are fundamental to a child's health and development, and they also maintain the space for the adult teeth to grow into.

Question: What happens if a baby tooth comes out too early?

Answer: Baby teeth (dentists call them primary or deciduous teeth) aren't just for chewing. Each one also acts as a guide for the permanent tooth that replaces it. If a primary tooth is lost too early, the permanent tooth loses its guide and can drift or erupt incorrectly into the mouth. Neighboring teeth also can move or tilt into the space, so the permanent tooth can't come in. Primary teeth can be lost too early for several reasons: They can be knocked out in a fall or other accident; Extensive decay can require that a primary tooth be extracted; Primary teeth can be missing at birth; some diseases or conditions can contribute to early tooth loss. If your child loses a primary tooth before the permanent tooth is ready to come in, or if the permanent tooth is missing, your dentist may decide to use a space maintainer. The space maintainer keeps the space open until the permanent tooth comes in.

Question: What are space maintainers, and are they really necessary?

Answer: Space maintainer are designed to maintain the open space left behind by the premature loss of a baby tooth, so that the adult tooth will be able to erupt into that space properly. Space maintainers can be made of steel and/or plastic, and can be made to be either removable or fixed in place. These devices can have an artificial tooth to fill in the space in more esthetic areas. Not every tooth that is lost requires a space maintainer. Usually if one of the four upper front teeth is lost early, the space will be maintained on its own until the permanent tooth comes in. Your dentist will periodically take an X-ray to follow the growth progress of the adult tooth. When it is ready to erupt, the space maintainer will then be removed.

Question: What can be done to address the large space (diastema) between my child's front teeth?

Answer: This gap or space, (aka diastema) most often occurs between the two upper front teeth. It is normal to have this diastema during some stages of dental development. The space eventually closes after the permanent canine teeth (eye teeth) erupt into the mouth. However, in some people, the space does not close. If that is the case, orthodontic treatment may become necessary. If this gap is caused by an overly large frenum (thick gum tissue above and between your front teeth) then orthodontic treatment would not be effective here. In that case a frenectomy (removal of that tissue) would be indicated to allow the teeth to come together again. If the large space is due to undersized lateral incisors (the teeth next to the two front ones) then bonding, crowns or veneers may become indicated to help close the gaps.

Question: Why do some teeth grow behind another? What should be done when that happens?

Answer: Teeth are normally supposed to grow beneath the tooth it is replacing, as to slowly cause the roots of the baby teeth to be resorbed as the adult teeth grow in. As the roots are being resorbed, the baby teeth will start to loosen and come out on their own. On occasion, the adult teeth will grow in differently, usually towards the inside of the mouth when this happens. If the second set of teeth are growing inside of the teeth they are supposed to replace, then the first set would need to be removed by your dentist in order to create the space needed to allow for the adult tooth to grow into the right position. In most cases the tongue will naturally guide the tooth into the correct position. In some cases, when there is too much crowding, interceptive orthodontics may become necessary to help create the space necessary for the adult teeth that are growing in.

Question: What are peg laterals?

Answer: Peg laterals are your top lateral incisors (the teeth on either side of your upper front teeth) which on occasion, can grow in peg shaped form. It is an anomaly that happens in about 5% of the population. Peg-shaped upper lateral incisors tend to be hereditary to some extent. It is often referred to as microdontia, which means teeth that are smaller than normal. Usually this condition is bilateral (occurring on both sides of the mouth). However, occasionally, an upper lateral incisor can be missing on one side and peg-shaped lateral present on the other side.

Question: What should be done to treat a peg shaped tooth (peg laterals)?

Answer: Individuals with peg-shaped lateral incisors can have bonding, veneers or crowns placed over or around this smaller tooth to create the illusion of proper shape and proportion. Typically, it is recommended to do bonding until the patient's jaw and teeth stop growing, and then place a more permanent restoration, such as a veneer or ceramic crown, once the growth has ceased.

Question: How many people are born missing one or more of their adult teeth?

Answer: The failure of one or more teeth to develop (partial anodontia), is an anomaly that occurs in a small percentage of the population. The most common teeth to be congenitally missing are the third molars (wisdom teeth), lower second premolars, and the upper lateral incisors (in that order). In fact, there is about a 25% chance that someone will not develop one or more of their wisdom teeth. Additionally, the congenital absence of a baby tooth is not common. However, if this were to occur, it is most likely the upper lateral baby incisor that is missing. In these cases, when a baby tooth is not present, it becomes highly unlikely that its permanent replacement will develop as well.

Question: How many people are born with extra teeth?

Answer: Extra teeth (referred to as supernumerary teeth), occur approximately 2% of the time in the adult set of teeth, and less than 1% in the child's first set of teeth. Most of these extra teeth (about 90%) will occur in the upper arch of teeth (maxilla). Supernumerary teeth may also be referred to as polydontia or hyperdontia, with the most common type being the mesiodens (an extra tooth that tends to form between and just inside of the upper two front teeth. Most of the time, these extra teeth don't even come through the gums, and they are discovered when taking an x-ray in that area. Other types of supernumerary teeth include the rare fourth molar (also referred to as paramolar or distomolar). Multiple supernumerary teeth are very rare in people that don't have any syndrome or disease associated with it. It is more common to be missing certain teeth, than to develop extra teeth.

Question: My dentist told me I have a double tooth. Why does this happen, and is there any way to make it appear more like a normal, single tooth?

Answer: A double tooth, or joined tooth occurs in one of a few ways.

- ❖ **Fusion** – where two separate teeth are attached together, sharing the dentin and enamel (the inner and outer layer of tooth structure) and often sharing the pulp chamber (where the nerves of the tooth are located) as well. The roots are separate.
- ❖ **Gemination** – is when you have what appears to be two teeth developing from a single tooth germ, sharing the pulp chamber and the root. When you count the teeth, it would still appear that you have the correct number of teeth, unlike fusion, where the count would be reduced.
- ❖ **Concrescence** – is different than germination in that the joining of tooth roots by cementum (the outer layer of the root) occurs after tooth formation is complete. This condition doesn't have much clinical significance unless you need to have the tooth extracted. If this were to become necessary, careful examination of the X-rays would be very important.

There are ways to make a fused tooth appear to be more like a single tooth. This may involve some reshaping of the enamel, some bonding to add better anatomy, and sometimes the use of porcelain veneers to create the individualized appearance.

Myth vs. Fact

Myth: It is okay to let my children brush their own teeth.

Fact: This will depend on the child. While it is great to build up a child's self-confidence and independence, children do not usually develop the full coordination and understanding of what they are trying to accomplish until the age of 6 or 7. Even though they may want to do this all by themselves, it is recommended that the parent or guardian supervise, check, and when necessary, do additional brushing for their child at least up until the age of 10. Your toddler can have their toothbrush available for "pretend or play" tooth-brushing along with you. Cavities prevented during this time will save a lot of time, money and trauma in the future.

11

GERIATRICS (ELDER CARE)

Fun Fact...

The average human produces enough saliva
in their lifetime to fill 2 swimming pools.

Important information for those getting long in the tooth

*"A person's greatest accomplishment
in their lifetime is how many people
they have touched with their smile"*

People are living longer and longer. At the turn of the 20th century the average age one could be expected to live was about 47 years; one hundred years later, the average life expectancy soared to 78 years. The majority of the elderly generations are now living healthy and active lifestyles. Today, more of the older adults have their own teeth and fewer dental restorations due to the improvement in home care, hygiene practices and preventative dentistry. In fact, many older adults are expressing their desire to enhance the esthetics of their mouth by having their teeth whitened and their smile made over. However, there are many challenges associated with getting older, including complex medical conditions, numerous medications, physical and mental debilitations, etc. As their motor control becomes compromised, and their motivation to diligently care for their oral health diminishes, numerous problems can arise and present a challenge for their dental care provider. Due to the high correlation between maintaining proper oral health and one's health in general, it becomes increasingly more important to practice good home care and maintain proper oral hygiene.

Geriatric (Elder Care)

Question: What is geriatric dentistry?

Answer: Geriatric dentistry involves the delivery of dental care to older adults, and involves the diagnosis, prevention, and treatment of problems that are associated with the normal aging process and its age-related diseases. With all the advancements in medical care, people are living longer, and more care is needed to preserve their dentition as they age and experience various pathological conditions and disabilities.

Question: What are the dental complications associated with the aging process?

Answer: The physiological changes that are associated with growing older can affect every aspect of the body. The cardiovascular system doesn't adapt as well to the stresses imposed on it, and the arteries can thicken causing an increase in blood pressure. As a result, the cardiovascular system of an older individual is more likely to develop cardiac ischemia (a restriction in blood supply), arrhythmias (abnormal heart rhythms) and heart failure. Skeletal changes also occur, such as osteoporosis, which is characterized by a decrease in bone mass and an increase susceptibility to fractures. This increased fragility and decreased bone mass can prevent one from being a good candidate for implants to replace failing or missing teeth, and the loss of bone mass can make it more difficult for dentures to fit comfortably. Elderly patients can develop a decreased flow of saliva causing a dry mouth (xerostomia), which impacts dental care in numerous ways, including an alteration or loss of taste, difficulty swallowing, tooth decay, yeast infections, gum disease, bad breath, and burning sensations in the mouth. Often times, the medications that they take to combat their illnesses will have an additional drying effect on the mouth making things that much worse.

Geriatric patients undergo many central nervous system changes such as memory loss (amnesia) and confusion (Dementia and Alzheimer's Disease). Depression is also very common as we age due to a host of potential factors including social isolation, loss of loved ones, physiological changes and psychological factors. Additionally, their immune systems become more compromised, therefore, becoming more susceptible to viral and bacterial diseases.

Other dental considerations, to keep in mind, include as one gets older, the nerves within the teeth recede, causing diminished sensory levels in their teeth, which results in the elderly seeking care for their cavities at a much later date since they were less aware. Their soft tissues are also much more frail than they used to be and they heal slower. The incidence of oral cancers increases as one ages as well.

Question: What are the difficulties associated with geriatric dental home care?

Answer: One of the most common difficulties associated with dental home care among the elderly population is the onset of arthritis. An individual with painful arthritic conditions in their hands will have difficulty holding a toothbrush and maneuvering properly. There are special brushes that are sold with better handles that are more comfortable to grip. Additionally, an electric brush may be better suited to remove the plaque and food debris, since they are more effective with less effort. Flossing could also be very difficult, and there are special floss holders with an ergonomically designed handle that are easier to use. A geriatric patient may also need to increase the frequency of their recall visits from every 6 months to every 3 months.

12

ORAL SURGERY

Fun Fact...

During the middle ages, people went to barbers for tooth extractions. These practitioners were called barber surgeons and were marked by the iconic red and white striped barber poles that we still see today.

It's like pulling teeth...

"Be true to your teeth, so they won't be false to you."

Oral and maxillofacial surgery is a dental specialty that exists to correct a wide variety of diseases, injuries and abnormalities in the hard and soft tissues of the head, neck, face and jaws. It includes, but is not limited to: wisdom teeth removal, apicoectomy, correcting TMJ disorders, facial trauma, corrective jaw surgery, oral pathology, dental implants, anesthesia and bone grafts. Oral surgery is a practice that has been around for centuries, dating back to the times of Hippocrates and Aristotle. Centuries later in France, barber surgeons became a common trade, where barbers not only cut hair, but performed extractions as well. In the 1700's the surgeon dentist was recognized, and a century later the oral surgery specialty became established.

Today, oral and maxillofacial surgeons have years of advanced technology and research to assist them in performing state-of-the-art procedures in a predictable fashion. Things that were not possible yesterday may soon be possible tomorrow. Implant dentistry, to replace missing or lost teeth, may now be considered to be one of the greatest advancements in dentistry today. However, this technique may become outdated by the regeneration of teeth through stem cell growth in the near future. It is truly exciting to know that every year something new is being introduced that can improve or change someone's life.

Oral Surgery

Question: What does an oral and maxillofacial surgeon do?

Answer: An oral and maxillofacial surgeon (oral surgeon) is someone who is well trained to correct a wide variety of diseases, defects and injuries in the head, neck, face, jaws and the hard and soft tissues of the oral and maxillofacial region. Oral surgeons have attended four years of dental school and at least four years of a hospital surgical residency program. They are specially trained to place dental implants, address TMJ (temporomandibular joint) disorders, handle various types of facial pain, and perform restorative surgical procedures such as bone grafting, sinus lifts, apicoectomies and wisdom teeth removal (both erupted and impacted). Oral surgeons specialize in addressing facial injuries, such as broken jaws, and are trained to treat oral cancers. An oral surgeon also has advanced training in anesthesia, so they can make your experience as painless and comfortable as possible. If your general dentist feels that a tooth extraction or other oral surgical procedure is more complicated or outside of their comfort zone, they will refer their patient to an oral surgeon.

Question: What does it mean to have an impacted wisdom tooth (third molar)?

Answer: Wisdom teeth usually erupt into the mouth between the ages of 17-21. Even when the wisdom teeth are fully formed, not everyone's wisdom teeth grow in (impacted), and some only grow in partially (partially impacted). Sometimes a person's jaw doesn't grow large enough to accommodate the growth of the wisdom tooth (third molar from the midline of the face), and other times the tooth develops on its side and will not erupt.

Question: When is it recommended to remove the wisdom teeth?

Answer: It is generally recommended to remove the wisdom teeth when:

- ❖ they are partially erupted, as this can leave an open communication for bacteria to enter and cause an infection
- ❖ they are growing in such a way that they can damage adjacent teeth
- ❖ if a cyst (fluid-filled sac) forms, destroying surrounding structures such as bone or tooth roots

Question: Can wisdom teeth cause your teeth to crowd as they grow in?

Answer: People who notice that their teeth are crowding as their wisdom teeth are growing in, may be blaming the wrong culprit. This crowding tends to happen at this age (late teens to early 20's) whether or not the patient has wisdom teeth. This crowding may also occur whether or not that individual had braces too. Often times teeth tend to crowd because of a late growth of the lower jaw coupled with a flattening of the profile of the face. Of course, the lack of compliance with wearing their retainer after orthodontic treatment may also be the source of this crowding, resulting in a relapse of the original crowding.

Question: What is a sinus lift procedure, and when is it necessary?

Answer: In order for an implant to be successful and predictable, it needs to be placed in an area with adequate bone surrounding it.

Surgeons prefer the minimum height of bone to be 7mm and the width to be at least 5mm, in order to have successful integration of bone and adequate support and strength. When the patient doesn't have enough bone; certain procedures can be performed in order to make that patient a better candidate, such as bone grafting and sinus lifts (sinus augmentation). For patients who need to have teeth replaced in the back part of the upper jaw, many times the floor of the sinus is in the way, preventing the placement of an implant in that area. The oral surgeon can augment the sinus by lifting the sinus membrane and filling in the base of the sinus with bone grafting material to give more vertical height. For example, if an 8 mm implant needs to be placed, but there is only 4mm of bone beneath the floor of the sinus, after the sinus is lifted and bone is placed, they can now get at least 4mm of extra bone for its successful placement. This procedure takes place at the oral surgeon's office and begins with a local anesthesia to the area being worked on.

Question: What is bone grafting, and where does the bone come from?

Answer: Bone grafting is the placement of bone within and around certain areas that are deficient in bone or have some defects that could compromise the placement of implants and affect function and esthetics in the mouth. The best source of bone for your graft is your own bone tissue from elsewhere in your body, because it is the most biocompatible and offers faster healing times when compared to other methods. However, it is not always the most practical or desired, since this bone would usually involve a procedure that takes some bone from your chin, the back of your lower jaw, the hip or your tibia. In many cases, a combination of artificial bone substitutes and freeze dried, demineralized, sterilized cadaver bone is used. The grafted bone provides an anchor and allows the existing bone to integrate with it, providing an environment suitable for the placement of implants.

Question: What would happen if I just left the space after the oral surgeon extracts my posterior tooth?

Answer: The loss of a back tooth can affect your dental health, your physical appearance and the way you chew, speak, sing and smile. When a tooth is lost, the adjacent teeth may tilt towards that empty space, or the teeth in the opposing jaw may drift up or down towards that space. Tipped teeth are more difficult to maintain, and are therefore more prone to decay. In addition, the surrounding bone and gum tissues may break down, resulting in an increased risk for gum disease. You may find yourself favoring the opposite side of your mouth when you chew, causing additional stress to your teeth and gum tissues. The loss of a tooth may also result in the failure to maintain the natural shape of your face, due to the lack of lip and cheek support in that area. The outcome may be an older appearance due to a sinking of your mouth in the region where the tooth was lost. Missing teeth can and should be replaced. Speak to your dentist to explore the many options you have, including implants and fixed bridges, which come very close to duplicating the function and appearance of your natural teeth.

Question: How soon can one exercise after minor dental surgery like a tooth extraction, gum surgery, apicoectomy, root canal, etc.?

Answer: There is no definite answer for everyone. As a general rule, do not perform heavy exercise for at least one or two days after your swelling has subsided. This may wind up being a week or until your stitches come out, but use common sense or ask your dentist if you have any questions. Exercising too early after surgery will make bleeding more likely. Rest, sleep, proper care and attention at home are important for the wound to heal properly. You have to listen to your body before you restart your exercise regimen. You may resume your normal activities the next day, but just do not engage in vigorous exercise such as heavy lifting, competitive sports, running, biking, etc.

Myth vs. Fact

Myth: My wisdom teeth aren't bothering me, so I don't need to have them removed.

Fact: Wisdom teeth don't always need to be removed. Some people's mouths are large enough to accommodate their growth, and others have wisdom teeth that don't come close to erupting. However, there are many times when wisdom teeth should be evaluated for removal even in the absence of any form of discomfort, in order to prevent possible cysts, infections or impact on the adjacent teeth.

13

ORAL CANCER, LESIONS AND GROWTHS

Dental Fact...

> 25% of oral cancer victims do not use
> tobacco or alcohol products and have
> no other lifestyle risk factors.

No joke here. What you need to know:

"Early detection and diagnosis can make a tremendous difference in one's life expectancy"

While the overall incidence and death rates of cancer has decreased over the years, recent studies by the American Cancer Society have indicated that oral cancer has actually increased. One person dies every hour from oral cancer in America alone, with a death rate higher than that of that of cervical cancer, Hodgkin's disease, cancer of the brain, liver, testes, kidney, and ovary. Even though smokers are 6 times more likely to develop cancer, 25 percent of oral cancer victims never even used tobacco products. The main reason oral cancer has such a high mortality rate is because, more often than not, it is detected in its later stages. When oral cancer is detected early, it can be curable 90 percent of the time.

Just as Pap tests, mammograms and colonoscopies are readily accepted by patients to help rule out and detect some of the more common cancers, oral cancer screening exams need to become a routine and accepted part of all dental exams. Today's oral cancer screening technologies can improve the accuracy of the exam, help determine whether biopsies are necessary, and save the lives of those whose cancers are caught early.

Oral Cancer, Lesions and Growths

Question: Who is at risk for oral cancers?

Answer: Most people are surprised to learn that each year one person dies every hour from oral cancer, making this type of cancer deadlier than cervical, brain, ovarian or skin cancer. In fact, recent statistics published by the American Cancer Society estimates that while the incidence and death rates for cancers overall have decreased, new cases of oral cancer and deaths associated with oral cancer are increasing. We know that early detection tools such as Pap smears, PSA tests and mammograms have greatly reduced death rates for cervical, prostate and breast cancers. Since oral cancer is one of the most curable diseases when caught early, it is extremely important to see your dentist regularly to keep your mouth under surveillance. When premalignant lesions or early stage oral cancers are found, treatment is simpler, less invasive and more than 82 percent successful. In continuing efforts to try and provide the most advanced technology and highest quality care available to patients, dentists are continually including new and improved types of oral cancer screening exams as an integral part of their regular examinations.

Question: What are the warning signs for oral cancer?

Answer: The two types of lesions that could be the precursors to cancer are white lesions (called Leukoplakia) and red lesions (called Erythroplakia). The red lesions are less common, but they have a much greater potential to become cancerous. If a red or white lesion does not resolve itself within 2 weeks, it should be reevaluated and a biopsy should be considered for a definitive diagnosis. Other possible signs and symptoms of oral cancer include:

❖ Difficulty in chewing or swallowing
❖ Numbness of the tongue
❖ Hoarseness
❖ Ear pain
❖ Difficulty when moving the tongue or jaw
❖ A lump or a thickening of the soft tissues in the mouth

If any of the above symptoms last for more than two weeks, a thorough exam and any necessary lab tests would become indicated.

Question: What are the risk factors for oral cancer?

Answer: The risk factors for oral cancer include: tobacco and alcohol use, exposure to sunlight (especially for lip cancer), age (incidence of oral cancer rises steadily with age), gender (men are twice as likely as women to get oral cancer), and race (African Americans are twice as likely as Caucasians to get oral cancer). Note, of all the risk factors tobacco is the primary cause of oral cancer, which accounts for 90% of all cases. Smokers are 6 times more likely to develop oral cancers than nonsmokers.

Question: How can you lower your risk for oral cancer?

Answer: Most oral cancer is preventable. Approximately 75% of oral cancers are related to the use of tobacco and alcohol. If you are among those using both, your risk becomes much greater than if you were using each substance alone. In order to decrease your risk you should avoid the use of any tobacco products (including cigarettes, chew, pipes, cigars and snuff), minimize the amounts of alcohol that you take in, use an SPF lip balm to protect from sun exposure, and eat plenty of fruits and vegetables to help reduce your risks.

Question: What can be done to detect oral cancers?

Answer: With oral cancers, the earlier the detection the greater the prognosis. Oral cancer is known to spread fairly quickly, with only half of those diagnosed surviving more than 5 years. Your dentist should incorporate or request your permission to perform an oral cancer screening exam each year as part of their office protocol. If they don't offer you the exam or perform this task, you should request the exam or seek care elsewhere. The exam should include an overall evaluation of the face, lips head and neck, with a thorough inspection of the inside of the upper and lower lips, the gums, the inside of the cheeks, the floor of the mouth, the tongue (the sides, top and underside), and the roof of the mouth. Newer types of oral cancer exams include tests that use fluorescent lights and special rinses and dyes (such as Toluidine Blue) to help dentists spot abnormal changes in the mucous membranes that line the inside of the mouth and throat.

Question: What are some of the benign (non-cancerous) ulcerative lesions that we may find in the mouth?

Answer: Among the most common, benign ulcerative lesions are:

❖ **Aphthous Stomatitis** (also known as the common ulcer) – is the most common type of oral ulceration that affects about 20% of the regular population, with 50% prevalence in those individuals experiencing some form of psychological stress. These lesions begin as reddish areas that develop into a whitish-yellow area with a red halo. The number of lesions may vary from one to hundreds, and can be quite painful for 10-14 days. Treatment includes topical antibiotics, antiseptic rinses, and dietary supplements. Sometimes topical corticosteroids are required to help resolve the symptoms and limit their recurrence.

❖ **Traumatic Ulcers** – as the name suggests, are ulcers that are caused by some form of trauma to the superficial layers of the soft tissues in the mouth. They can arise from dental injections, biting the cheek, tongue or lip, or getting poked by a sharp crust of bread or a chip, etc. They are usually seen on the tongue, lips or inside of the cheeks. They can present as a painful, single lesion with a reddish border and a yellow, pus-like center. This area will heal on its own, but can be made to feel more comfortable by using topical numbing agents or rinses.

❖ **Herpes Simplex** - There are two strains of the herpes simplex virus, Type I (HSV-1) and Type II (HSV-2). HSV-1 is the type that is associated with the lips, mouth and face and transmitted via saliva, while HSV-2 is usually sexually transmitted. HSV-1 is the most common type of herpes virus, and many people develop the related sores (lesions) inside the mouth, such as cold sores (fever blisters). HSV is never eliminated from the body, but stays dormant and can reactivate, causing symptoms. When the virus is active, painful ulcerations can develop, but the main indicator of a primary infection is from seeing a diffuse, reddish and painful gum inflammation. Multiple pinhead reddish ulcers tend to cluster and join together over several days. It is normal to experience fever and enlarged lymph nodes during this time. Diagnosis is usually made by labs tests of the cells and tissue. Treatment of the primary infection includes fever reducing medications and fluid management. Antiviral medications such as acyclovir will help to lessen the duration and severity of the lesions. There is no known cure for HSV infection, but treatments can reduce the likelihood of the virus spreading and manifesting itself.

❖ **Acute Necrotizing Ulcerative Gingivitis (ANUG)** – also known as Trench Mouth, as this disorder was common among the soldiers during World War 1. Stress and a diminished resistance most often bring about ANUG. Other factors that cause it include: smoking, poor oral hygiene and inadequate nutrition. It is a painful infection with crater-like ulcerations, swelling, sloughing off of dead tissue from the mouth, and accompanied by a bad odor from the area. Fever, enlarged lymph glands and malaise (general discomfort or uneasiness) are sometime present too. Treatment includes cleaning out the bad tissue, followed by an antibacterial rinse such as chlorhexidine or dilute hydrogen peroxide.

Additionally, rest, proper diet, nutritional supplements, and proper home care along with abstaining from smoking, alcohol and spicy foods are advised.

❖ **Lichen Planus** – Oral lichen planus is a chronic autoimmune inflammatory condition that can affect the lining of your mouth, and usually manifests as scattered, white, pinhead elevations that are interconnected by white lines to appear like lacy white patches. Oral lichen planus occurs most often on the inside of your cheeks but also can affect your gums, tongue, lips and other parts of your mouth. Sometimes oral lichen planus can involve your throat or esophagus. An initial episode of oral lichen planus may last for weeks or months, but it is usually a chronic condition that can last for many years. Although there's no cure at this time, this condition can be managed with medications and home remedies.

Myth vs. Fact

Myth: I don't smoke so I can't get oral cancer.

Fact: It has been established that tobacco is the primary cause of oral cancer, which accounts for 90% of all cases. Smokers are 6 times more likely to develop oral cancers than nonsmokers. However, even non-smokers can get oral cancer. The risk factors for oral cancer, aside from tobacco, include: alcohol use, exposure to sunlight (especially for lip cancer), age (incidence of oral cancer rises steadily with age), gender (men are twice as likely as women to get oral cancer), and race (African Americans are twice as likely as Caucasians to get oral cancer). While smokers fall into the highest risk category, it is highly recommended that everyone be screened routinely for oral cancers.

14

MEDICAL CONDITIONS (AS IT RELATES TO YOUR DENTAL HEALTH)

(Sub categories: Autism, Cancer, Diabetes, Heart Disease, Herpes, Multiple Sclerosis, Pregnancy, Tobacco Use)

Dental Fact...

Regular dental cleanings can
help prevent heart attacks.

The link between the mouth and body

*"The majority of systemic diseases
have oral manifestations"*

Each year we are learning more and more about just how closely linked our mouths are to the rest of our body. New studies continue to demonstrate the impact of gum disease on various medical conditions such as diabetes and heart disease. Conversely, we are also learning about how certain medical conditions such as pregnancy, autism, multiple sclerosis and cancer can affect the health of our mouths and the way we care for them. We see how various stresses that affect our minds and bodies can affect our mouths and initiate lesions such as herpes. Additionally, tobacco addiction, which is considered a disease, not a habit, can affect both the body and the mouth in many detrimental ways. This section explores the most frequently asked questions in the way many of these medical conditions relate to the mouth.

Medical Conditions that can affect dental health and treatment

Autism

Question: What is autism?

Answer: Autism is a severe developmental brain disorder that usually manifests within the first 3-4 years of a child's life. Children that are affected by this disorder tend to have difficulty with their communication, language, behavior and social skills. Although children with autism may appear normal, this developmental disorder specifically affects brain function in the areas that are responsible for the development of appropriate social interaction skills and communication.

The incidence of autism is about 1 out of every 110 people; this disorder is more common in males than females (4:1 ratio). Although its cause still remains largely unknown, autism is a lifelong condition. While most children with autism demonstrate normal physical health, this disorder can be affected by both genetic and environmental factors. Early diagnosis and intervention is paramount, as it could significantly improve the child's communication and social behavior later in life. Educational and behavioral therapy is the most important thing you can do for an autistic child, along with a lot of love and patience.

Question: What are the early signs and symptoms of autism?

Answer: Symptoms and behaviors of those diagnosed with autism vary from each individual, with each child displaying a unique set of behavioral traits. Early symptoms include:

- ❖ Lack of eye contact with mother by 12 months of age
- ❖ No response when baby's name is being called by mother
- ❖ A baby appearing to be deaf
- ❖ A baby resisting when being held by mother

- ❖ Not saying single words by the age of 16 months
- ❖ No two word phrases by 24 months

Question: What are some of the ways to recognize children with autism?

Answer: Children with autism may display any combination of the following behaviors:

- ❖ Approximately 50% of autistic children are non-verbal
- ❖ They often run away from their caretakers
- ❖ They may appear to be stubborn
- ❖ They may exhibit rambling speech
- ❖ They may perform self-stimulating behavior such as rocking back and forth or flapping their hands
- ❖ They may not respond to you
- ❖ They may not be able to answer easy questions
- ❖ They may display a sensitivity to light, sound, touch and odor
- ❖ They may develop a seizure (usually occurs in 25% of affected children)

Question: How does having autism affect one's dental care in the office?

Answer: New experiences can become a problem for those individuals with autism. Loud noises, such as a dental drill, may irritate the autistic patient. Bright lights may be disturbing and affect behavior; sunglasses may need to be supplied. Certain smells, tastes or textures may become upsetting. The autistic patient may not be comfortable being touched by the dental professional, or tolerate the movement of the chair. It is important that their appointments be short and prompt so that they are not kept waiting. Additionally, the autistic patient may have difficulty communicating the location of their discomfort to the dentist, and may respond to any discomfort in an unusual way.

Question: What can be done to improve the chances of a successful dental visit for an autistic patient?

Answer: First, you should contact the dental office to make them aware of any special needs, and to arrange a visit and tour of the office to help make the autistic patient more comfortable with the staff and their surroundings. Use photos, books and toys to help familiarize the patient. By preparing and explaining what is going to happen, you will help instill confidence. Make sure that the patient is accompanied by someone they know well, and encourage them to bring any items, toys or favorite videos that will help comfort them during their visit.

Second, remind the dentist team to ease into any procedure, and to try and avoid sensory overload and sudden movements. The first visit should be a short, quiet and positive appointment. Good behavior should be praised and poor behavior ignored. Everything should be explained and demonstrated before it is done, such as showing the instruments that will be used. Your dental provider should speak calmly and positively, and have the patience to tell the patient where and why they need to touch them with a piece of equipment. Since autistic patients tend to take everything more literally, it is important that they be addressed in specific, short sentences.

Question: How does having autism affect one's teeth and gums?

Answer: Pediatric gastroenterologists have found that children with autism tend to regurgitate their food and the stomach's acids more than once a week, causing the teeth to erode. The dentist should also check the teeth for signs of bruxism (grinding), since this is evident in about 20 to 25 percent of children with autism. Additionally, many of the medications used to treat the various aspects of autism can have adverse dental side effects, which can affect swallowing, speech and the use of removable appliances due to a decrease of salivary flow.

Cancer

Question: What are the side effects of cancer therapies such as chemotherapy and radiation therapy on the mouth? What special precautions should one take?

Answer: Side effects in the mouth from chemotherapy or from radiation to the head and neck can be very serious, as these therapies not only kill cancer cells, but may also harm normal cells, including those in your mouth. Complications common to both types of therapy include: painful mouth and gums, ulcerations, rampant decay, dry mouth, burning sensations in your tongue, change in taste, and difficulty eating, talking and swallowing. Suffering individuals are also more likely to develop infections, which can delay or force the cessation of cancer treatment.

The most important piece of advice that you could recommend to any person diagnosed with cancer is to visit their dentist at least two weeks before starting their chemotherapy or radiation therapy. The dentist will perform a complete exam, take all necessary films, and address all mouth problems before they can become a possible source of infection or decay.

Individuals who develop dry mouth are more prone to tooth decay due to the decreased levels of saliva that they can produce. Fluoride rinses are not enough to prevent the tooth decay that can occur from the dry mouth caused by the chemotherapy or radiation therapy. Instead, a fluoride gel placed inside a custom-made mouth tray is recommended. In order to minimize the harmful effects of dry mouth, one should avoid sugary substances such as candy or soda (unless sugar-free), chew on ice chips, sip water frequently, suck on sugar-free candy, or chew sugar-free gum to stimulate salivary flow.

Many times, as a result of cancer therapy, people develop jaw stiffness and a limited opening of their mouth. To prevent this, exercise the jaw muscles three times a day by opening and closing the mouth as far as possible, (without causing pain), 20 times. Results are best after using warm, moist compresses or by performing the exercises in a warm to hot shower.

Other beneficial recommendations include brushing the teeth, gums and tongue gently, using an extra-soft toothbrush that had its bristles softened in warm water. Floss gently everyday, but stay clear of those areas that are sore or bleeding. Avoid using toothpicks, tobacco products and alcohol. Stay away from hard, crunchy or spicy foods that can irritate your mouth. Avoid alcohol-containing mouth rinses, but rather use a baking soda and salt solution (1/4 teaspoon of baking soda, 1/8 teaspoon of salt in 1 cup of warm water) followed by a plain water rinse. Even if cancer therapy has started, you can still make sure that the oncologist works in a team approach with the dentist.

Diabetes

Question: What is the link between diabetes and gum disease (periodontal disease)?

Answer: More and more studies are showing a link between the mouth and the rest of the body regarding the spreading of infections. Over 400 different types of bacteria can exist in the human mouth. Many of them thrive in sugars, including glucose, the sugar linked to diabetes. Persons with diabetes have greater than normal risk of gingivitis (inflammation and bleeding of the gums) and periodontal disease, the condition that causes millions of people to lose their teeth. Like any infection, gum disease can make controlling the blood-sugar level very difficult. Diabetes can cause the blood vessels to thicken, in turn slowing the flow of nutrients and the removal of harmful wastes. The result is weakening the resistance of the gums and bone tissue to the spread of infection. Researchers have found that diabetes predisposes a patient to gum disease. Moreover, recent evidence strongly suggests gum disease can worsen the severity of one's diabetic condition.

Many diabetic patients with severe cases of gum disease struggle to maintain their normal blood-sugar levels, and as a result their need for insulin increases, infections originating in the mouth can easily spread, and may enter the bloodstream. In cases of severe gingivitis and periodontal disease, even the simple act of brushing or flossing can introduce bacteria into the bloodstream, aggravating health troubles in other areas of the body. Experts expect that treatment of periodontal disease may diminish fluctuations of blood-sugar levels, along with a decreased risk of diabetic retinopathy (damage to the retina that could lead to blindness in diabetics) and the associated risk of damage to the arteries.

People with diabetes are also at risk for developing thrush, a yeast infection in the mouth that causes white spots on the tongue. This infection thrives on high glucose levels in saliva. Another oral manifestation found in uncontrolled or undetected diabetics is dry mouth (xerostomia), an ailment that may result in halitosis (bad breath). Smokers are five times more likely to develop gum disease. A smoker with diabetes age 45 or older is 20 times more likely to get severe gum disease.

If you have diabetes, make certain to inform your dentist and book a visit for an examination and cleaning at least every six months. You should schedule your dental appointments for about an hour and a half after breakfast and after you have taken your diabetes medication. Try to arrange shorter visits, preferably in the morning.

Heart Disease

Question: What is the link between heart Disease and gum disease (periodontal disease)?

Answer: If your doctor were to say your cholesterol levels were too high and you had double the chance of developing heart disease, would you do something about it? Most people would. They may consult a nutritionist, start an exercise regimen or simply modify their diet by eliminating cheese or switching to egg whites. Now suppose you discovered the incidence of heart disease was twice as high in people with periodontal disease, and you were one of the millions of people who suffered from this condition. Would you set up an appointment with your dentist? According to some studies, periodontal disease (which affects the bone and tissue surrounding your teeth) has proven to be a stronger risk factor than any of the other conditions usually linked to heart disease (i.e. hypertension, high cholesterol, age and gender). Oral bacteria can infect damaged hearts and certain oral bacteria can cause platelets to aggregate. New findings have emerged to explain how and why bacteria that cause periodontal disease can also increase the risk of heart disease. Researchers at Harvard's School of Dental Medicine and presenters at the 150th annual meeting of the American Association for the Advancement of Science also concluded that the bacteria found in plaque (the primary etiological factor causing gum disease) is linked to coronary disease. People with periodontal disease are up to two times as likely to suffer a fatal heart attack and nearly three times more likely to suffer a stroke as those individuals without this disease. It is speculated that oral bacteria, the most common form being streptococci, enters the bloodstream through small ulcers in the gum tissue. The bacteria cause the platelets in the bloodstream to aggregate and form blood clots (thrombi) that can block blood vessels and infect heart valves.

When you consider the effects of gum disease, think not only in terms of how it affects your teeth, but also how it could possibly lead to a serious and perhaps fatal infection from the release of bacteria into your bloodstream. Avoid other risk factors such as smoking and chewing tobacco, both of which have a detrimental effect on the severity of the gum disease. Systemic diseases like diabetes can lower the oral tissue's resistance to infection, making periodontal disease even more severe. Review your medical history with your dentist. Many of the medications or therapeutic drugs that you may be taking can decrease your salivary flow and adversely affect your teeth and gums. Prevention is the key to success. Teeth are intended to last you a lifetime, and a healthy heart and body should help improve your overall quality of life.

Herpes

Question: What is herpes?

Answer: There are two strains of the herpes simplex virus, Type I (HSV-1) and Type II (HSV-2). HSV-1 is the type that is associated with the lips, mouth and face and transmitted via saliva, while HSV-2 is usually sexually transmitted. HSV-1 is the most common type of herpes virus, and many people develop the related sores (lesions) inside the mouth, such as cold sores (fever blisters).HSV is never eliminated from the body, but stays dormant and can reactivate, causing symptoms. When the virus is active, painful ulcerations can develop, but the main indicator of a primary infection is from seeing a diffuse, reddish and painful gum inflammation. Multiple pinhead reddish ulcers tend to cluster and join together over several days. It is normal to experience fever and enlarged lymph nodes during this time. Diagnosis is usually made by lab tests of the cells and tissue. Treatment of the primary infection includes fever reducing medications and fluid management. Antiviral medications such as acyclovir will help to lessen the duration and severity of the lesions. There is no known cure for HSV infection, but treatments can reduce the likelihood of a virus spreading and manifesting itself.

Multiple Sclerosis

Question: What is MS (Multiple Sclerosis)?

Answer: Multiple Sclerosis (MS) is a progressive, degenerative neuromuscular disorder that often results in partial or full paralysis, with no known cure. Remissions, both complete and partial, are common. This disorder causes the demyelination (the removal of the fat-like protective sheath that surrounds the nerves and protects them) of the nerves of the central nervous system (CNS). This can result in the following: a decrease in the speed of nerve conduction, partial blocking of the nerve conduction, a modification in the way nerve impulses are transmitted, or a complete failure of transmission for these nerve impulses.

Those individuals diagnosed with MS are particularly susceptible to suffering from unnecessary pain and treatments as a result of not recognizing the impact that MS can have on their oral health care. Preventative dental care and procedures can tremendously improve the oral health and lives of people with this debilitating disorder.

Question: How does having MS (Multiple Sclerosis) affect your dental care in the office?

Answer: Patients with MS can have their good days and their bad days. While minor cases of MS may not impact one's dental care, severe MS requires special considerations when seen in the dental office. Patients with severe MS should have shorter dental appointments, preferably scheduled in the mornings. If a longer appointment is necessary, 5-10 minute breaks should be taken every half hour. Patients with MS should be seated at a 45-degree angle to avoid compromising their airway. Individuals with MS can develop respiratory problems, since the disease affects the muscles that control their breathing. It may be indicated to use a rubber dam, as long as the patient can breathe well through their nose. It can also be hard to maintain the mouth in an open position for extended periods of time. For this reason a mouth prop may be used to help the mouth remain open comfortably.

Patients with MS may also be unable to pinpoint the source of their pain or discomfort, so great care is required to diagnose dental problems before committing to root canal therapy or extractions. Sometimes individuals with MS can develop trigeminal neuralgia (a nerve pain disorder in the face where episodes can be triggered by a touch to the face) on one or both sides. Temporary numbness in the teeth, jaws and lips may be reported. Multiple Sclerosis may also result in partial or total paralysis of the face, causing dental procedures to become more challenging.

Additional considerations include: wheelchair access (if the disease becomes so debilitating) and some form of general anesthesia or sedation (either in the office or in a hospital).

Question: How does having MS (Multiple Sclerosis) impact one's homecare?

Answer: Patients with Multiple Sclerosis may develop difficulties swallowing, using their tongue properly, and producing enough saliva. As a result, it becomes increasingly more difficult for these individuals to maintain proper dental home care and will therefore have a greater chance of developing cavities and gum disease. Since people with MS have compromised dexterity from the loss of control of their muscles, brushing and flossing can become very difficult. Special types of modified brushing and flossing aids are available (check with your dentist and pharmacy), and caregivers are encouraged to assist with the home care when appropriate. Additionally, various medications (such as immune-suppressant drugs, corticosteroids, muscle relaxants, and antidepressants) tend to dry out the mouth, accelerating the development of cavities and gum disease. Keeping the mouth hydrated, salivary substitutes and fluoride treatments are often recommended.

Question: Are there any types of dental treatment that should be avoided with individuals that have MS (Multiple Sclerosis)?

Answer: Patients who have more advanced stages of MS may have a lot of difficulty wearing full or partial dentures. First, since individuals with MS are more prone to developing a dry mouth, it will become increasingly more difficult to eat, talk, and wear their dentures. Second, the muscle spasticity makes wearing theses removable appliances very difficult and sometimes dangerous when the symptoms of MS become severe. In order to avoid these issues, one may consider placing dental implants that can anchor and support the denture, minimizing its chance of dislodging.

Question: Is it possible to mistake early signs of Multiple Sclerosis for TMJ problems?

Answer: Multiple Sclerosis (MS) can cause a variety of different symptoms depending on which nerves are attacked. While it may be possible that MS can affect the area where the TMJ dysfunction was diagnosed, it is more likely that the two are unrelated. To make the right determination, one should seek the care of a neurologist who specializes in treating patients with MS. Treatment should be coordinated with a dentist who is comfortable diagnosing TMJ disorders.

Pregnancy

Question: What special considerations should be given to the pregnant patient when they undergo dental care?

Answer: The goal of dental care during pregnancy is to provide the necessary services without causing any adverse effects to the mother or the developing baby. Any extensive or elective treatment should be postponed whenever possible. However, avoiding necessary treatment would be unwise, and potentially carry greater risk than the risk associated with the procedure. For example, if there is a large area of decay present close to the nerve, and this cavity can potentially cause an infection that could be harmful to you or your baby, it would make sense to address this problem as soon as possible (with clearance from your obstetrician). It is recommended that the pregnant patient have at least one cleaning during their pregnancy to minimize the chance of developing pregnancy gingivitis (inflammation, bleeding and swelling of the gums that are heightened in response to the plaque due to the hormones associated with pregnancy). Fluoride supplementation is recommended starting around the third month of pregnancy, since this is when the baby teeth start to mineralize.

It is recommended that X-rays should be avoided during pregnancy, unless it is essential that one be taken to help address a dental emergency. If an X-ray needs to be taken, a second lead vest should be used to help cover the abdominal area. Additionally, the dentist should take care to avoid using local anesthetics containing epinephrine (a vasoconstrictor) and drugs that can cross the placental barrier. Tylenol is usually considered to be fine by most obstetricians for controlling discomfort. Penicillin and Erythromycin are usually considered acceptable antibiotics when the risk of an infection outweighs the risk of taking these medications. Check with your obstetrician first before starting any type of medication. Anxious patients should avoid taking barbiturates, anti-anxiety medications (such as valium) and nitrous oxide when pregnant.

Question: How should you stage dental care when pregnant?

Answer: Except for emergency care, only preventative dental treatment and hygiene appointments should be carried out during the first trimester. The best time to provide dental care is during the second trimester, since most of critical systems of the body have matured to the point where the risk to the fetus is less likely. Dental treatment can proceed into the third trimester if the patient is comfortable.

Tobacco Use and Vaping

Question: What is the link between tobacco use and gum disease (periodontal disease)?

Answer: We all are getting to be very familiar with the link between the use of tobacco, lung cancer and heart disease. Did you know that tobacco could wreak havoc in your mouth, from bad breath to oral cancer? Compared to nonsmokers, smokers are many times more likely to develop gum disease, larger deposits of tartar on their teeth, cavities (due to a drier mouth) and eventual tooth loss (from periodontal disease). Smoking can also act to delay healing after surgical procedures or tooth extractions. In addition, smoking has also been shown to be detrimental to the successful integration of implants. Recent studies have identified cigarette smoking as a major independent risk factor for periodontal disease (the disease that affects the bone and tissue surrounding your teeth).

Research has shown that when variables such as oral hygiene, age, gender, systemic diseases, medications, and frequency of dental visits are controlled, cigarette smoking is the strongest predictor for developing periodontal disease. Smokers tend to develop gum disease at earlier ages and have more severe cases of it. Research has found that cigarette smoking more than doubled the rate of tooth loss for an individual, and increased the possibility of becoming completely toothless by 4 times.

When a smoker is in need of periodontal therapy, a deep dental scaling tends to not result in significant reduction of pocket depths. In addition, surgical gum therapy does not usually result in longstanding reductions of pocket depths in patients who smoke. Smokers tend to respond poorly to gum therapy and heal much slower than non-smokers.

The Centers for Disease Control and Prevention (CDC) have conducted several comprehensive studies; the most recent data indicated that smokers were 4 times as likely to develop gum disease, and former smokers were 1.7 times more likely, than non-smokers. For current smokers, there is a dose dependent relationship between cigarettes smoked and the likelihood of developing periodontal disease. For example, if someone smoked 9 cigarettes or less per day they were 2.8 times as likely, whereas if they smoked 31 or more, the odds increased to almost 6 times as likely to develop periodontal disease.

Cigarettes not only affect the teeth and their surrounding structures, but they act to suppress the immune system, decreasing one's ability to fight off infections and diseases. Most people are surprised to learn that each year one person dies every hour from oral cancer. Approximately 75% of these cancers are attributed to the use of tobacco (primarily cigarette, pipe and cigar smoking) when combined with alcohol. When alcohol is combined with tobacco, the risk for oral cancer increases by more than 15 times. It has been well documented that the use of tobacco increases the prevalence and severity of periodontal disease and subsequent tooth loss. Recent studies have shown that more than 50% of the cases of periodontal disease that affects our nation's adult population may be attributable to cigarette smoking.

Smokeless tobacco users are 4 times more likely to develop oral cancer than non-users. Chewing tobacco and snuff are the two main categories of smokeless tobacco. Their use has been well established as a cause of oral cancer. Tobacco is considered to be the single most significant initiator of the development of oral squamous cell carcinoma.

It has been estimated that over 100 billion dollars are spent each year on direct medical care for smoking-related illnesses. This seems a bit outlandish considering that tobacco is the single most preventable cause of disease and death in the world. Despite increased public awareness and tobacco-cessation products, a large percent of the population still smokes, and many more are involuntarily subject to second-hand smoke. The Surgeon General's report stated, among its major findings, that "Lifestyle behaviors that affect general health, such as tobacco use, excessive alcohol use, and poor dietary choices, affect oral and craniofacial health as well."

Historical Summary of the Surgeon General's Reports on Oral Health and Tobacco:

- Since 1964, oral cancer and tobacco have been linked. Evidence relating pipe smoking and lip cancer established.
- Effects of tobacco on gingivitis, periodontal disease, nicotine stomatitis identified in 1969.
- Alcohol found to work synergistically with tobacco reported in1980
- By 1986 all types of tobacco products - cigars, cigarettes, pipes and smokeless tobacco - were implicated in the development of oral cancer.

The dental profession, as a whole, has become increasingly more aware of the detrimental health effects of tobacco, and has begun to take measures to stop its use. Recent surveys are showing that dentists are becoming involved in tobacco-cessation activities, and many feel that it is their duty to encourage and assist their patients to end or at least limit their tobacco use. Dentists are also in a good position to help prevent the initial or continued use of tobacco by children and adolescents through positive anti-tobacco messages. The dentist should advise the teen or young adult to quit, citing reasons that include: reduced athletic ability, mouth odors, and stained teeth, in addition to educating them on the risks of lung cancer, oral cancer and heart disease. Since people tend to visit their dentist more regularly than they see their physician, the dentist should accept the role of the primary educator on the harms of tobacco use.

Question: What are the effects of vaping on oral health?

Answer: Vaping (smoking e-cigarettes) has become a very popular replacement for cigarettes with the thought that it would become a healthier alternative to tobacco and a safer way to quit smoking. The bottom line, according to more and more research, is that vaping can be just as dangerous, if not more dangerous, when compared with smoking, and these e-cigarette companies are adding flavoring products to attract and appeal to the younger population. Early studies on vaping show that it can impact the health of the lungs, damage blood cells, increase the risk of heart disease and negatively impact one's immune system.

The dangerous effects of nicotine have been well established. Nicotine acts in a way that reduces the blood flow to the gum tissue, since it is a vasoconstrictor, and that, in turn, restricts the amount of oxygen and nutrients needed to keep the gums healthy and not cause the gum tissue cells to die and thereby recede. Since vaping can affect the immune cell function and decrease connective tissue turnover, there is a much greater chance of developing gum disease, tooth sensitivity, cavities and potentially tooth loss. Although the percentage of nicotine is much lower than in traditional tobacco products, one electronic cartridge (200 - 400 puffs) can equal the harmful effects of smoking 2 - 3 packs of regular cigarettes. Studies have shown that the nicotine inhaled through vaping may increase one's risk of cancer (especially lung, gastrointestinal, pancreatic and breast cancers) by damaging the DNA. However, the vapor not only contains nicotine, which is bad for the teeth and body on its own, but also has ultra-fine particles of toxic chemicals and heavy metals. Many of these chemicals are linked to not only cancer, but also to respiratory disease and heart disease. Additionally, since nicotine is a stimulant, it may have some indirect effects on the mouth, such as causing one to more readily clench and grind their teeth, which can contribute to teeth sensitivity, cracking and fracture.

Vaping works by heating a liquid comprised of propylene glycol, glycerin, water, flavoring and nicotine or THC. Propylene glycol, when used orally has been shown to be very harmful to the tooth's enamel and surrounding gums. Vaping often causes xerostomia (dry mouth), which significantly reduces the amount of saliva produced and can thereby contribute to more plaque build-up, increased bacteria, the development of more rampant decay, bleeding and swollen gums, periodontal disease and other oral health issues. It is important to note that a diminished salivary flow, resulting in a dry mouth, is also one of the main causes of bad breath (halitosis).

Myth vs. Fact

Myth: Smoking can't cause your teeth to fall out.

Fact: Smoking can wreak havoc in your mouth. Smokers are many times more likely to develop gum disease, larger deposits of tartar on their teeth, cavities (due to a drier mouth) and eventual tooth loss (from periodontal disease). Smoking can also act to delay healing after surgical procedures or tooth extractions. In addition, smoking has also been shown to be detrimental to the successful integration of implants. Recent studies have identified cigarette smoking as a major independent risk factor for periodontal disease (the disease that affects the bone and tissue surrounding your teeth). In fact, the research has shown that when variables such as oral hygiene, age, gender, systemic diseases, medications, and frequency of dental visits are controlled, cigarette smoking is the strongest predictor for developing periodontal disease. Smokers tend to develop gum disease at earlier ages and have more severe cases of it. Research has found that cigarette smoking more than doubles the rate of tooth loss for an individual, and quadruples the possibility of becoming completely toothless.

15

FEAR, ANXIETY AND PAIN CONTROL

Dental Fact...

People with dental phobias have a higher risk of gum disease, early tooth loss, and poorer health in general.

Take three deep, cleansing breaths and read on

"With the right person, in the right environment and with the right amount of patience and encouragement you can overcome anything"

Fear of the dentist is not innate, it is a learned behavior. Fear and anxiety develop out of socialization and personal experience. Additionally, the mass media will often communicate misinformation, and cause inaccurate perceptions that will contribute to one's anxiety.

The right dentist, with understanding, patience, compassion, and a gentle touch should be able to convert an anxious, scared patient into a loyal, non-fearful patient. The wrong dentist may say negative remarks or perform certain actions that contribute to the patient's fears. A sizable portion of the general population who could benefit from dental care does not receive treatment because of fear. Some people will wait until the pain they have is enough to exceed the avoidance tendency. During this time small problems can develop into much larger issues.

Trusting the dentist is a major issue. The most reliable and most powerful means of reducing one's fear and anxiety is through direct positive experiences with a dentist. The patient's renewed trust in their dentist and the inter-personal relationships they develop will help pave the way for much more enjoyable dental visits. Often times the most fearful of dental patients can become the dentist's biggest fan once their fears and anxieties are alleviated.

Fear, Anxiety and Pain Control

Question: Why do some people have a fear of dentistry?

Answer: People are not born fearful. Fear and anxiety develop out of socialization, personal experience, and the mass media (movies, television, news stories, etc.). Newspaper and magazine cartoons, along with comedy sketches also are guilty of misinformation, and create inaccurate perceptions that contribute to one's anxiety. Fear can come from an individual's own personal perception of the situation, which is usually based on past experiences coupled with their interpretation of the present situation.

A sizable portion of the general population who could benefit from dental care does not receive treatment because of their fear. What produces the most fear is the sound of the "drill" and the "needle." They may be terrified when they sit in that big chair, but as soon as the dentist makes them numb, they are so relieved, that they sometimes fall asleep. They discover almost immediately that the dental injections are not very painful. It's just that there is a tendency for patients to concentrate on the stimulus of the injection, and by doing that they magnify that stimulus into something much more unpleasant than it should be.

Question: What is the difference between fear, anxiety and phobia?

Answer: Fear is the individual's emotional response to a perceived threat or danger.

Anxiety denotes an emotional experience similar to fear, but where the source of threat is ill-defined, ambiguous, or not immediately present. Phobia is a special form of intense fear recognized by that individual as excessive or unreasonable in proportion to the actual level of danger.

Question: How can a patient overcome their fear of dentistry?

Answer: Numerous studies have shown that the critical element is that the patient believes he or she has some sort of control over the potential threat. Therefore, if the dentist can convince the patient through words or actions that he or she can terminate the procedure if they feel the need (by raising their hand as a sign, for example), then less fear and less pain will likely be experienced. If the patient feels that they have no means of influencing treatment, then they may develop a perception of helplessness and lack of control, which fuels their fear.

Some apprehensive patients need to be told everything that is going to be done, so they know what to expect. (i.e. warnings when they may feel pressure or vibration, what they are likely to experience next, etc.) A lack of information may result in fear. By developing a sense of trust with their dentist, a once fearful patient can become the most dedicated and loyal patient.

Question: How can one cope with their fear and anxiety once they are in the dental chair?

Answer: Coping skills include learning to relax and breathe properly, utilizing distraction techniques, and asking questions to gain control. Sometimes candles, waterfalls, relaxation music, headphones, television, movies, etc., will enable the patient to relax more. Additional ways of controlling fear and anxiety is by administering Nitrous Oxide (laughing gas), oral premedication (i.e. Valium, Ambien, and Xanax), IV sedation, and giving pain free injections after using a strong topical numbing agent. Of course, having a dentist and staff that is patient, understanding and comforting is the most important factor in helping to cope with one's fears and anxieties.

Question: How can you prevent a child from developing a fear of dentistry as they grow older?

Answer: Factors contributing to a positive outlook on dentistry involve early encouragement and positive communication by parents, and a relatively pain-free experience with a dentist who communicates with the patient, treats them with respect, and allows the patient to have some say in their treatment, if they desire. Starting kids early, by two years old, and making the visits fun with magic tricks, balloon animals, toys, counting teeth, brushing the teeth models, seeing their teeth on the TV screen, playing fun music or allowing them to watch their favorite shows or movies can really make a difference. These kids will develop a positive association with the dentist and look forward to future visits. Never use the dentist as a threat if they don't brush or if they eat too much candy. If you make the dentist out to be the bad guy, the children will carry that thought with them throughout their adult life.

Question: What can happen as a result of avoiding dental care?

Answer: What starts as a small cavity can become very serious, if left untreated. Some people wait until the pain they have is enough to exceed their avoidance tendency. This fear of pain is one of the major reasons why patients fail to seek help from a dentist until their emergency becomes too severe. At that point, what should have been a simple cavity now becomes a more involved root canal or extraction. Additionally, a patient who avoids routine dental cleanings and gum maintenance can wind up with severe gum disease (periodontal disease), which causes gum recession, bone loss, tooth mobility and the eventual loss of teeth. Swellings and infections may result from neglecting these cavities and gum issues, and what would have been unnecessary costs and procedures will now be necessary to restore the mouth back to a better state of health and function.

16

DENTAL EMERGENCIES

Dental Fact...

An adult tooth that has been knocked out starts to die within 15 minutes, but if you put it in milk, or in your mouth's saliva, it will survive longer.

There is never a good time to have a dental emergency

"Avoiding proper dental care often turns a simple problem into a dental emergency"

A dental emergency can occur at any time. It can happen on vacation, eating a meal, during the night, while playing sports or during recreational play. It can affect you or your loved ones, and usually when you least expect it. Dental emergencies (such as a toothache, swelling or infection) can often be avoided with diligent preventative dental care. Emergencies that result from trauma may not be fully avoidable, but safety precautions such as sports mouthguard and supervised play can help minimize injuries. Of course, there is always that tooth that gets cracked or broken when biting into something hard, or the crown that gets pulled off eating something chewy. Dental emergencies can happen when you least expect it. Some may not make sense, such as the spontaneous appearance of certain lesions or sores, and bleeding that just won't stop after you've had oral surgery. Many of your questions and concerns will be answered and described in this chapter.

Dental Emergencies

Question: What should I do if there is a dental emergency?

Answer: The most important thing you should do is to try and remain calm. Understand that injuries to the mouth, teeth and face do happen frequently with both adults and children. In order to minimize the traumatic situation and comfort the injured person you must remain calm and take the appropriate prompt action. The next thing you should do is to assess whether or not the accident involved hitting the head or causing them to lose consciousness at all. If consciousness was lost, even briefly, then you should contact a physician immediately, and then focus on the teeth once everything is stabilized. If there is any bleeding, use a clean towel or gauze, and then check around you for any broken or missing teeth. It is possible broken fragments may have entered parts of the lip. If any teeth are missing, you should look for them in case they can be utilized.

Question: What should I do if my child's baby tooth gets knocked out (dental avulsion of a primary tooth)?

Answer: The first thing you should do is contact your child's dentist as soon as possible. The baby tooth ***should not*** be replanted because it may cause subsequent damage to the developing permanent tooth. Usually this type of injury happens between 7-9 years of age, when the bone surrounding the tooth is softer and more resilient. This means there is less of a chance of a bone fracture around the tooth. Your dentist should then see your child to check and verify that everything else is fine.

Question: What should I do if my child's adult tooth gets knocked out (dental avulsion of a secondary tooth)?

Answer: The first thing you should do is try to find the tooth and put it in a cup or baggie with your own saliva, milk or saline, (to keep it hydrated), and bring it immediately to your dentist. *Do Not Touch the root of the tooth; handle it by its crown.* **Time is of the essence**! With each minute that passes, the chance of reattachment becomes less and less. *DO NOT SCRUB* the tooth! If you do it will wipe away its outer ligament and prevent its reattachment within your empty tooth socket. If you are in a place where dental care is not accessible, then gently rinse it in cool water, (no scrubbing or using soap), only if there is dirt on it, (otherwise leave it alone), and slowly replace the tooth within the socket immediately and hold it there with gauze. Remember, the faster you act, the better your chances of saving the tooth. Almost all replanted teeth will show some signs of root resorption and ankylosis (where the root fuses with the surrounding bone). It is possible that this may affect one's bite later on.

Question: What should you do when a tooth fractures or gets chipped?

Answer: If a tooth sustains a fracture or chip from a traumatic accident, you should contact your dentist immediately for an X-ray and evaluation. Keep the mouth clean and if there was any trauma to the lip you should apply cold compresses to reduce swelling. If you cannot find any broken tooth fragment, check the lips to make sure the fragment didn't get embedded in that area. Simple chips can be smoothed or repaired with tooth-colored bonding. A more serious fracture may require root canal therapy, (if the nerve is involved), or extraction, (if the fracture happens along certain areas of the root surface). Moderate fractures may be bonded for now, and later restored with crowns, veneers or onlays. For children, you should try to hold off on these more advanced restorations until your child has completed their growth.

Question: What causes a toothache?

Answer: A toothache occurs when the nerve within the tooth gets damaged or inflamed. This problem is usually caused by bacteria from tooth decay communicating with the nerve of the tooth. Cavities (tooth decay) are usually brought about by a combination of poor oral hygiene coupled with eating a lot of sticky, sugary and starchy foods. These bacteria feed on the sugars and starch left over from poor brushing and flossing. As a result, acids are produced that will slowly eat away at the good tooth structure until the nerve becomes damaged, causing the toothache. Another way the nerve can get damaged is from dental trauma (i.e. sports injury, rough play or fights, severe teeth grinding, or extensive dental work on hypersensitive teeth).

Question: What are the symptoms of a toothache?

Answer: The signs and symptoms of a toothache include: lingering sensitivity to cold (that persists even after the stimulus is gone), sensitivity to hot, spontaneous and constant throbbing pain, discomfort or pain when chewing or touching the tooth, swelling or tenderness around the area that hurt, and possibly fever as well.

Question: What should I do if a severe toothache develops?

Answer: Prescribed or over-the-counter pain medication, (dosed for children according to weight and age), may temporarily quiet the symptoms. In case the toothache is originating from the gums, rinse with warm salt water and floss the teeth to remove any food or substance that may be stuck between the teeth or in the gum pocket around the tooth. Antibiotics may become necessary; however, it is recommended that you contact your dentist to help make that determination. Once seen by the dentist, an examination and X-rays should be performed to verify damage and to help determine the treatment. A comprehensive medical and dental history should also be taken. Upon discovery, the decay and/or affected nerve tissue may be cleaned out and replaced with a sedative or permanent filling. If there is an abscess (pus-filled swelling), it may need to be drained. If the tooth is not restorable, an extraction may become necessary

Question: What should you do if you tell your dentist that you have tooth pain, but after taking an X-ray nothing is found to be wrong?

Answer: An X-ray is only one tool that is used to help diagnose a problem. They are 2-dimensional images that may or may not lend a clear picture as to what is going on. Sometimes, if an X-ray is taken from a different angle, more information can be detected. When teeth overlap in a picture, cavities can be missed. If an X-ray is over-exposed (darker) or under-exposed (lighter) it may not reveal what needs to be found. If X-rays are taken at the wrong angle the teeth may appear longer or shorter than they are and distort the picture. If an X-ray does not reveal any information to help your dentist determine your pain, then other diagnostic tests must be performed, including:

- ❖ Percussion (tapping the tooth)
- ❖ Palpation (feeling the gums around the tooth)
- ❖ Pocket depth probing (to measure the pockets around the teeth for gum problems)
- ❖ Checking occlusion (to see if your bite needs to be adjusted)
- ❖ Testing for fracture of the tooth or cusp of the tooth
- ❖ Hot and cold sensitivity tests (indicating if the nerve is damaged)
- ❖ Pulp Tester (an electronic measure of nerve vitality)
- ❖ Checking for sinus problems that can masquerade as tooth pain
- ❖ Checking other areas for referred pain (pain originating from another area)
- ❖ Determining stress levels and possible teeth grinding and clenching
- ❖ Clinical exam (performed by the dentist to evaluate the complaint)

If an X-ray and all the above tests still don't explain why you might have developed your discomfort, do not lose hope. Sometimes it may take a while for the true cause to manifest. Follow-up consultations and exams may be necessary before the cause becomes clear.

Question: What should be done if a jaw fracture or severe trauma to the head is sustained?

Answer: If this should happen you must seek medical attention immediately. A severe head injury can be life threatening, and facial fractures may block the air passage and affect your breathing. Keep in mind that an emergency medical team will most likely reach you faster than you can get to the hospital. Facial fractures usually involve the lower jaw, but may also include the upper jaw, cheeks, eye sockets or nose. For children, their bones are still somewhat soft and the fractures are usually incomplete and heal quickly with few complications. If you suspect the jaw may be fractured, stabilize the jaw with a necktie or towel around the head. Do not allow it to move. Apply cold compresses, and go to an oral surgeon or hospital emergency room immediately.

Question: What precautions can I take to prevent dental injuries from occurring?

Answer: The risk of dental injuries can be greatly reduced by doing the following: First, make sure that protective athletic gear, including a sports mouthguard, is worn to prevent severe injuries to the mouth. Second, check to see that you and your child are properly secured in the car, using the appropriate car seat or seatbelt. Third, be aware of your surroundings, and prevent unnecessary injuries at home by taking precautions and childproofing the house for younger kids. And fourth, advise your children to avoid rough play and to not run fast in confined or slippery spaces. Note that many traumatic injuries occur from 18 to 40 months of age, because this is a time where your uncoordinated toddler is learning to walk and run.

Question: What should I do if my child's tooth gets displaced outward, inward or to the side (luxation), pushed up (intruded) or pushed down (extruded)?

Answer: After assessing the injury, making sure your child is conscious and breathing well, contact your child's dentist for immediate evaluation. For toddlers, the most common type of tooth displacement is a luxation, because the bone around the baby teeth is very soft, and teeth can move more easily within the socket. When this happens, there is usually a lot of bleeding from the surrounding gums. During a fall, a child's tooth is usually pushed inward, towards the palate. This is less damaging to the developing tooth bud because as the crown portion of the tooth moves inward, the roots are pushed away from the developing tooth. The most damaging type of displacement is intrusion (when the tooth is pushed upward), because the root of the baby tooth can be forced into the developing tooth bud, causing possible developmental issues and color changes with the developing adult tooth. If the baby tooth is pushed up less than 3mm, it has an excellent prognosis and chance of re-erupting on its own. This would allow the baby tooth to spontaneously erupt over a 2 to 3 month period - as long as the developing adult tooth bud is not injured. If re-eruption does not begin within 2 months, the baby tooth will need to be removed. If the baby tooth is pushed up more than 6mm, the tooth is hopeless. If the baby tooth is displaced into the developing adult tooth, it should be extracted to prevent further damage to the adult tooth bud. It is very important to take an X-ray to see if the tooth is present, because a severely intruded tooth may be pushed all the way inside and appear to have been knocked out.

If an adult tooth gets displaced, gently try to reposition the tooth back into the right place if possible and hold the tooth in place and seek immediate dental care. If a tooth gets displaced less than 5mm, there is a 50% chance that the nerve won't be damaged. These teeth may reposition themselves, but may also require orthodontic repositioning. It is possible that there could be a fracture of the bone surrounding the tooth during these luxations. If the tooth is very loose, and can be moved more than 2mm, a flexible wire and composite splint may be placed for 7-10 days to help stabilize it.

Question: What should be done for a laceration (cut) inside the mouth?

Answer: All lacerations within the mouth must be cleaned well and checked for any foreign bodies. A tongue laceration usually requires stitches if the edges of the tissue does not line up cleanly. Any tears to the frenum (muscle attachments) will usually heal well, without any long-term complications. Use icepack to minimize swelling, and give the appropriate pain medication if necessary.

Question: What does it mean when a tooth turns dark or discolored?

Answer: Discoloration or the darkening of a tooth usually results from a tooth that has been traumatized from an injury that caused damage to the nerve. This discoloration usually happens 2-3 weeks after the accident. If the tooth turns dark after an injury, it is because the blood supply got damaged. Baby teeth usually do get lighter over time, (about 6 months on average), and if the tooth doesn't bother him/her you can leave it alone. Usually the color change bothers the child's parents more because of the esthetics. Adult teeth are handled differently. If an adult tooth changes color, that implies that the nerve inside is dying, and root canal therapy will be indicated. An adult tooth that shows no signs of color change after an accident may still turn color in the near or distant future. Your child's dentist should keep monitoring the tooth for change and any signs of any infection. A pink tooth indicates either internal resorption (where the internal aspects of the tooth start to resorb), or the presence of blood pigments within the tooth. The pink tooth needs to be monitored closely.

17

PREVENTATIVE CARE

Dental Fact...

The second most common disease, after the common cold, is tooth decay.

Prevention: A little goes a long way

"Avoid trouble by not getting into it in the first place"

There has been a shift in the way children's dental care is now approached. Instead of waiting for dental problems to arise (such as their first cavity, or cross-bites and crowding) and then intervening to address and correct the problem, we are now taking a more preventative approach with early intervention.

For many years after fluorides were introduced, the incidence of cavities had been on the decline. The combination of parents becoming complacent as a result of this dental trend, coupled with the fact that often times both parents are working, and extended family or caretakers are being placed in charge of the child's home care, is resulting in dental cavities back near their all time highs. With the availability of electric brushes, fluoride rinses, dental sealants, digital X-rays and other cavity detecting technologies, we have the ability to help prevent the onset of these cavities. Starting children's dental visits at an early age, preferably before any dental issues have had a chance to arise, will help foster better relationships with the dental providers and contribute to a positive association with their dentist. Having regular check-ups will enable the dentist to recommend ways to prevent dental problems from arising in the near or distant future. This preventative care will ultimately wind up saving money, time and aggravation over time.

Preventative Care (Sub categories: Sealants, Fluorides, X-rays)

Sealants

Question: What are dental sealants?

Answer: Dental sealants are tooth-colored or clear shaded resin (plastic) materials that are applied and bonded to the chewing surfaces of the back teeth in order to fill in the pits and grooves of the teeth making them easier to clean, (by making the grooves more shallow and smooth), and creates a barrier that makes them less likely to develop tooth decay. Many adults and children have such deep grooves that the bristles of the toothbrush cannot reach fully to clean out the food and plaque. As this debris sits there, the acids and bacteria in the mouth continue to break down this food and make the enamel more porous and more likely to develop a cavity. Sealants fill in these pits and grooves so the brush can do its job more easily.

Question: Who is a candidate for dental sealants?

Answer: Both children and adults are candidates for dental sealants. Since children don't lose their baby molars until the age of twelve, it is important to protect these teeth from developing cavities and problems that can affect the developing adult teeth. Adolescents are very prone to developing cavities due to their dietary habits and poor home care, and the sealants can help to prevent decay in the grooves of the teeth that usually get passed over during a quick brushing. Any adult can benefit from sealants as well, making it easier for cleaning out the food and plaque, giving them an extra line of defense in the battle against tooth decay.

Question: How are sealants applied?

Answer: Each sealant only takes a few minutes to place. First, the teeth are cleaned well and checked to make sure that no decay is present. If there are any signs of decay in those grooves, then they must be cleaned out and filled with the sealant material or a filling material if deeper. Once the chewing surfaces are cleaned, they are roughened up with an etchant (weak acid solution), a primer and an adhesive to enable the sealant material to bond to the tooth enamel. The sealant material is hardened by a light source, operating at a certain wavelength, to set the material and make it solid.

Question: How long do sealants last for?

Answer: Depending on what type of material was applied, what types of food are being eaten (harder, crunchier foods can wear them down faster), and how good the home care is, sealants can last several years before they may need to be reapplied. Your dentist should be periodically checking to make sure that the sealants are still intact and serving their purpose. Reapplying the sealants will ensure that the tooth is protected against decay, and will save the expense of having a more involved restoration on that tooth in the future should cavities develop.

Fluorides

Question: Why is fluoride necessary?

Answer: Fluoride helps to prevent against tooth decay by strengthening the tooth's enamel and making it more resistant to acids and harmful bacteria. Fluoride can be administered topically to adults and children to help prevent against cavities and fluoride toothpastes and gels are also used to help control tooth sensitivity, especially when the roots are exposed due to gum recession and teeth grinding. When an individual is suffering from dry mouth (xerostomia), fluoride trays can be made to help prevent against rampant decay caused by a lack of salivary flow. A little fluoride is good for your teeth, but too much of it can lead to a condition called fluorosis, which can cause white spots on your teeth during the child's development.

X-rays

Question: Why are X-rays (radiographs) necessary?

Answer: Dental X-rays provide valuable information that your dentist could not detect otherwise. With the help of X-rays, your dentist can look at what is happening in areas that are not visible clinically. X-rays can detect cavities between the teeth, and can depict approximately how deep a cavity extends relative to the nerve. They can also help diagnose periodontal disease, abscesses, cysts, tumors, developmental abnormalities and infections in the bone.

Question: How often should X-rays be taken?

Answer: Typically every new patient should have a complete set of X-rays taken (about 18 films) to serve as a baseline. This set is taken every 3-5 years depending on the patient's needs and history. A set of 4 "bitewing" films is taken once each year to check for cavities between the teeth and to monitor their progression. A panorex X-ray is a film that is taken while you stand still and the X-ray head rotates around you, providing one solid film of your jaws and teeth. A panorex is recommended for children in order to evaluate their need for orthodontics, for teenagers and young adults to evaluate the growth of the wisdom teeth and decide if they need to be removed, and for adults of all ages to evaluate for possible cysts and abnormal growths. A periapical film refers to a single film that is usually taken whenever the dentist needs to evaluate a specific area of concern.

Question: Why do dentists need to take a new full set of X-rays every 3-5 years?

Answer: Routine X-rays help to prevent a small cavity from becoming a larger problem. Even if a patient is seen every 6 months, cavities can remain undetected between the teeth unless X-rays are taken periodically. Additionally, a comprehensive set of X-rays will show if an old root canal filling is failing, if there is periodontal disease (the breakdown of the surrounding tooth structures that involves bone loss), or if there is any decay recurring beneath the margins of older restorations, etc. A person who has a lot of old restorations in their mouth or is under dental care should have a full set every 3 years. A younger person with good home care and very few restorations and dental problems can have a full set every 5 years. It is still recommended though for a person to have their routine bitewing X-rays every year to check for the cavities that can develop in between the back teeth from not flossing.

There are many patients who refuse to take X-rays each time they come in, and then wonder how come all of a sudden their tooth, which recently started causing them discomfort, now needs a root canal or an extraction because the cavity has grown beyond the size of just a simple filling. If they allowed the dentist to take those periodic X-rays, then that lesion would have been caught when it was small, easy to fix, and less expensive to restore. Insurance companies usually allow a full set of X-rays to be taken every 3 years because they know it will become less expensive for them in the long run to reimburse for preventative care rather than crowns and root canals later on.

Question: How much radiation is in a traditional dental X-ray, and should I be concerned?

Answer: Typically the radiation considerations pose a far smaller risk than many undetected and untreated dental problems. Even so, all dentists should use a lead vest with a thyroid collar for extra protection. Each dental X-ray is about 0.5 mrem per film and a complete set is about 9 mrem. Just to put the amount of radiation into perspective, a barium enema: lower GI series is 875 mrem, and a mammogram is 500 mrem per breast. Note the average person gets about 360 mrem just from outside and background radiation (such as from foods and from outer space). In other words, you can have about 10,000 dental X-rays before you reach the maximum allowable amount per year. Note digital X-rays have even less radiation than traditional X-rays. Digital X-rays are about one tenth of the radiation from a traditional dental X-ray, which means you can have up to 100,000 digital X-rays to meet your annual quota and no one ever even comes close to that. A complete set, taken every 3-5 years, is only 18 digital X-rays. The radiation from a dental X-ray is negligible and the pros of taking it far outweigh any potential risks. So if you are really that concerned, then stay off your cell phone for a couple hours or avoid driving by the airport that extra time to make up for it.

Question: How are digital X-rays different than traditional X-rays?

Answer: Digital X-rays play an invaluable role in the diagnosis of dental problems. Digital X-rays eliminate many radiation worries because it requires 90% less radiation than conventional film X-rays. So a complete set of X-Rays (18 films) has the radiation of only 2 conventional films. It is as accurate as conventional X-rays and can even reveal things traditional films cannot. You can correct the contrast, and color-adjust the digital X-rays to reveal hidden problems. We can measure things more accurately and backlight teeth to see things that never could be seen with conventional film. Digital X-Rays are instantaneous. Once the sensor is exposed to digital X-rays the image is sent directly to the computer monitor for immediate viewing. So please allow your dentist to take the necessary digital X-rays to get the whole picture and make an accurate diagnosis.

Question: What are CBCT scans, what are their benefits and how much radiation do they have?

Answer: Cone-beam computed tomography systems (CBCT) are a variation of traditional computed tomography (CT) systems.

The CBCT systems used by dental professionals rotate around the patient, capturing data using a cone-shaped X-ray beam. The data is used to reconstruct a three-dimensional (3D) image of the patient's teeth, mouth, jaw, neck, ears, nose, and throat. Benefits of this type of imaging include providing a fast and non-invasive way to get answers to clinical concerns that a regular dental X-ray cannot. They are great for helping to determine the placement of implants, finding pathology, confirming failing root canals and detecting potential growths, etc. Dental CBCT scans typically only have about 10-20% of the radiation that other CT scans have. Dental CBCT scans also have less radiation than a complete set of digital dental X-rays because through the use of a cone shaped X-ray beam, the radiation dosage is lower, and the time needed for scanning is reduced. While a number of patients raise concerns over radiation, the clinical benefit of an X-ray imaging exam outweighs the small radiation risk.

18

NUTRITION AND DIET

Dental Fact...

Oral and systemic disease will occur less
frequently in a well-nourished body.

The importance of having a
strong, healthy foundation

*"A mouth that is kept healthy will
invariably lend itself to beauty"*

Nutrition and diet have a tremendous affect on your dental
health, playing a large role in the mouth's ability to resist infection
and develop gum disease. Any dental restoration will always have
a greater chance of long-term success when it is built upon a strong
and healthy foundation. Unfortunately, most people are nutritionally
deficient and choose diets that are not giving the body what it needs
to be healthy. There are some nutritional systems on the market,
such as **Isagenix®**, that have all the ingredients necessary to
support the health of your body and smile. Rather than reaching for
the junk food or eating whatever is in front of you, these systems
are inexpensive, easy to prepare, taste great and supply your body
with everything it needs to boost your immune system, release
unnecessary weight and build tone and strength.

The future of preventative dental care lies not only in proper home care, fluorides and sealants, but also in the prevention of disease through the consumption of a well-balanced diet and the necessary nutritional supplements. Many of the vitamins and minerals that our body needs have specific roles in the health of our oral structures from supporting healthy gums and strong bones and teeth to preventing infections and oral cancers. This chapter answers the most frequently asked questions regarding your diet and nutrition as it relates to your dental needs.

Nutrition and Diet

Question: What is the importance of diet and nutrition in dentistry?

Answer: Any dental restoration will invariably have a better long-term prognosis when built on a strong and healthy foundation. From a functional standpoint, inadequate nutrition will make the body, (including teeth and gums), more susceptible to gum disease, resulting in increased tooth mobility, bone loss, and eventual tooth loss. From a cosmetic standpoint, it is essential that restorations such as porcelain veneers and crown and bridgework be performed in a healthy mouth (free of gum disease) as red and inflamed gums can distract from the overall appearance. A mouth that is kept healthy will invariably lend itself to beauty.

Question: How does nutrition affect your smile?

Answer: It is very important not only to create the perfect smile, but also to make certain that perfect smile is built upon a strong and healthy foundation. The key to achieving this healthy smile is maintaining proper oral hygiene - regular dental check-ups, and taking nutritional supplements that are specifically geared towards optimum oral health. After all of the advances in dental office care and home care, 90% of the population is still developing periodontal disease. Nutrient deficiency can become a major contributing factor in periodontal disease by inhibiting the mouth's ability to resist infection. Nutrient deficiency can become a major contributing factor in periodontal disease by inhibiting the mouth's ability to resist infection, and eventually contribute to tooth loss. In other words - your diet does affect your dental health. The future of dentistry lies in the prevention of disease through the consumption of a well-balanced diet and the necessary nutritional supplements. Remember…disease will occur less frequently in a well-nourished body.

Question: How do I know if I have a vitamin and mineral deficiency?

Answer: The mouth is a mirror to the immune system. Unhealthy, bleeding gums are the first signs of a vitamin and mineral deficiency. The lack of magnesium, zinc, copper, manganese, selenium, vitamin E or vitamin C can allow rapid destruction of cell membranes, compromising the structural integrity of the cells, leading to gingivitis and periodontal disease. Bleeding gums attract scavenging bacteria, and the bacterial digestion of blood creates unpleasant mouth odors. It is a vicious cycle that can be quelled by proper oral hygiene, adequate diet and nutritional supplementation and the use of herbal remedies, as an adjunct to conventional therapies.

Question: Do most people have inadequate nutrition?

Answer: The USDA Food Consumption Survey reported that out of 21,000 people surveyed, not one consumed 100% of the RDA (recommended daily/dietary allowance) for ten key nutrients. These ten key nutrients included: vitamins B6, B12, A, C, thiamin, riboflavin, calcium, magnesium, iron and protein. Most people are blissfully unaware of the importance that vitamins play in a healthful lifestyle. According to an article written in the New York Times, only one in ten people (of the 12,000 people surveyed in ten states), have adequate diets. The US Public Health Service also found that 50% of the population was below the US RDA levels for one or more vitamin or mineral. According to the American Dietetics Association, only 20 to 30% of adults are consuming the recommended daily five or more servings of fruits and vegetables.

Question: What role do vitamins and minerals play in the mouth?

Answer: Vitamins and minerals play a major part in helping the body combat bleeding and swollen gums, loosening of teeth, tooth decay and halitosis (bad breath). Specifically, vitamins and minerals help form antibodies to fight bacteria and infection, boost the immune system, destroy foreign substances and eradicate toxins. Both vitamins and minerals share a symbiotic relationship. Vitamins cannot be used or absorbed without the presence of minerals. And our bodies cannot make minerals; we must ingest them through foods and supplements. Since most people tend to see their dentist more routinely than their physician, it is the dentist that can become the primary nutritional educator. In addition to regular brushing, flossing and routine dental check-ups, nutritional supplements can help to keep your mouth and body strong and healthy.

Question: What are the most common signs that someone has a vitamin and mineral deficiency?

Answer: One of the most common signs of vitamin deficiencies is an oral lesion - changes in the texture of the gums and lips and burning sensations of the tongue. Some of the oral manifestations of deficiency and metabolic disorders readily identified by dentists are: osteoporosis, diabetes, anemia, anorexia and bulimia.

Question: What role does folic acid play in the mouth?

Answer: Certain nutrients can help to prevent the defects brought about by their deficiency. For example, a recent study concluded that folic acid plays a vital role in the prevention of birth defects such as cleft lip and cleft palate during pregnancy. Additionally, women who may need more folic acid include frequent dieters, drug or alcohol users, smokers, women who take birth-control pills and women who consistently do not eat well-balanced meals.

Question: Do most people have inadequate diets?

Answer: Yes. Let's face it - most people do not eat well. Even bodybuilders, athletes and movie stars, (who look as if they are eating right), may not be getting all of the nutrition that they need. Findings indicate that unbalanced diets and subclinical deficiencies are becoming increasingly common. The majorities of individuals do not eat fresh vegetables, but would rather eat frozen, processed and canned vegetables. We are living in a society where children grow up on Big Macs® rather than a fresh, home-cooked meal, and where candy bars, instead of fresh fruit are the after school snack of choice. The results of these poorly balanced diets are evident in the mouths of our patients.

There are nutritional systems that have all the ingredients to support the health and beauty for your smile. These systems work synergistically to build and support your immune system; fuel the body's needs, boost your energy, release excess weight and increase your body's recovery time from all the rigors you impose on it. Additionally, cleansing can aid in accelerating the removal of these toxins and impurities from the body, while nourishing the body with vital nutrients to rapidly revive health. When toxins are released, the fat that binds to these toxins is more easily released as well.

Poor nutrition and a lack of certain key nutrients increase the risk of developing oral diseases, exposing the mouth to infection and periodontal disease. Periodontal disease is a condition that affects the majority of the population, and is the leading cause of adult tooth loss.

Approximately, 50% of all people have some form of gingivitis (inflammation of the gums), which is often a precursor to periodontal disease. Recent studies have shown that there is a direct link between periodontal disease and such serious conditions as heart disease and diabetes. Eating a well-balanced diet and taking nutritional supplements will help to strengthen one's immune system, promote healing and give individuals healthy teeth and gums.

In addition to periodontal disease, dietary deficiencies have been associated with such oral health conditions as: osteoporosis of the surrounding bone, loss of taste, bad breath and mouth and tongue sores. Deficiencies in vitamin C, iron and zinc could compromise the resistance of our gum tissue to the bacteria in dental plaque. So what recommendations should a dentist make to their patients regarding diet and nutrition? The number one suggestion is to eat a well-balanced diet and to take the necessary nutritional supplements; otherwise your teeth and gums may be at risk.

Question: Who has the greatest risk for inadequate nutrition?

Answer: Individuals who are at an even greater risk of developing nutritional deficiencies include smokers, diabetics, the elderly, adolescents, women during and after menopause and lactating and pregnant women. However, a poor diet is not the only reason people may be nutritionally deficient. Even if people are eating well, food processing, pollution, stress, alcohol, smoking and various medications and medical conditions can interfere with the absorption of essential nutrients or accelerate their depletion. Some of the drugs that prevent a person from receiving the benefits of a well-balanced diet include: aspirin, cold remedies, allergy pills, corticosteroids, laxatives, antacids, barbiturates, diuretics, caffeine and even birth control pills, illness, injury, physical and mental stress also place a strain on the body and act to deplete its nutritional stores.

Myth vs. Fact

Myth: I don't need to list the vitamins, minerals herbs and homeopathic remedies on my health history.

Fact: Dental health care providers should have the following questions on their medical/drug history form: "Are you taking any nutritional supplements?" and "Are you currently taking any herbal or natural homeopathic remedies?" and "If so, are you under the supervision of a nutritionist or an alternative therapist?" If these questions are not included on the form, then please make sure to tell your dentist, (and other doctors), exactly what you are taking. When taken appropriately, herbal and homeopathic remedies can have a wonderful healing effect on the body. Like many western drugs, herbal remedies have potential risks, side effects, and drug interactions that can interfere with traditional western medicines and affect the safe practice of dentistry. The Food and Drug Administration (FDA) currently regulates prescription and over-the-counter drugs but not herbal preparations. It is critical that you list any alternative medications and treatments so that your dentist can research the substance to see if there are any possible contraindications in order for you to be treated in a safe and effective manner.

19

HOME CARE

Dental Fact...

If you don't floss, you miss cleaning 35% of your tooth surfaces.

It's in your hands now

"It is not enough to have it... you have to use it"

Most people do not take proper care of their teeth. They wonder why their gums bleed when they brush and try to floss. They are told that they build up a lot of plaque and tartar, and become concerned when they hear that their gums and bone are receding and that cavities are developing in the areas between their teeth. The good news is that much of this can be corrected with proper home care. The bad news is that many people either are not taught how to care for their teeth properly or are too busy or lazy to execute their home care in the appropriate way. Most people brush inefficiently for less than thirty seconds with a manual brush, when they should be brushing for two minutes with an electric brush moving slowly around every surface of every tooth. Eighty percent of the population does not floss at all, unless there is something stuck between their teeth. Of those people that are diligent enough to floss, most are doing it wrong, which makes the act either ineffective or traumatic to the gums. Also, how many people are tongue scraping after brushing?

This chapter will address these topics and more; including discussions on how diet affects your home care, and the impact and use of other dental aids such as toothpastes, mouth rinses, etc.

Home Care

Question: What does proper home care mean?

Answer: Proper home care involves the combination of having an adequate diet, exercising proper brushing and flossing techniques, and utilizing additional adjuncts such as tongue scraping and rinses. A summary of these various facets of home care is summarized below:

Diet - Any food or snack that can become trapped within the pits and grooves of your teeth or between your teeth can become harmful if not cleaned properly. Chewy candy (i.e. taffies, caramels, jellybeans, and licorice) are among the biggest cavity culprits. However, you may be surprised to know that nuts, raisins and dried fruits can also cause a lot of damage, since they too get readily stuck in and around the teeth. The complex carbohydrates such as pretzels and potato chips get broken down into the same sugars that are found in cakes and cookies. Any food debris left on the tooth creates an acid attack in the mouth to break it down. The less likely the food is to dissolve or rinse away, the longer the acid attacks will be. Chocolate, which is full of sugar, is actually not as bad for your teeth as dried fruit and nuts, because chocolate dissolves quickly. However, you can prolong any acid attack by eating or drinking things slowly over a longer period of time. Additionally, if you can't get to a brush right away, you should rinse well with water, and can chew sugar-free gum for five minutes to help neutralize the acids in your mouth and lift out the debris from within the grooves of your teeth. This is especially important in those individuals with a dry mouth.

Brushing - It is recommended that everyone brush at least twice each day with a soft-bristled brush or electric brush. The first time should be in the morning, after breakfast, so your teeth are clean before leaving for school or work. It defeats the purpose of brushing if you eat a sugary vitamin after brushing, or nibble your breakfast on the go, because these substances will stay lodged in the top grooves of your molars and in between your teeth for hours to come, contributing to the formation of cavities. The most important time to brush is right before you go to sleep at night so that nothing is left on or in between your teeth when you are sleeping. The reason is that when you are awake, your saliva helps to bathe and rinse your teeth, but while asleep, you do not salivate that much, and your teeth are more susceptible to developing cavities from the debris left on them. Additionally, if you have the chance to brush after other meals or snacks, it would be advisable. Don't forget to brush your teeth after taking liquid or chewable medicines, as the sugars and acids contained in medicines may break down the tooth's enamel.

An electric brush has a few advantages over a manual brush. First it generates more brush strokes per second; making it more effective for the amount of time it is being used. Keep in mind that while it is recommended to brush for two minutes, the average person only brushes for thirty seconds. With an electric brush it is easier to clean behind the back teeth. Many of these electric brushes have certain extra bells and whistles such as a digital timer so you know when two minutes are up, and an indicator light to show if you are pressing too hard. There is usually less trauma to the gums and teeth when brushing with an electric brush since many over-zealous manual toothbrush users bang into their gums with the wrong technique, or scrub too hard. A manual toothbrush can be very effective with the right technique, and conversely, an electric toothbrush can be virtually useless with the wrong technique. If using a manual brush, use small, vibratory strokes on a 45-degree angle so that the bristles get in the pockets between the teeth and gums. Avoid the up and down or circular motion, as that can just traumatize the gums. If you are using an electric brush, try to spend at least two full seconds on each tooth surface (inside, outside and top), making sure to angle the brush between the teeth and having the bristles go between the tooth and the gums. Spin brushes are just a watered down version of an electric brush that may attract the attention of your child with its various themed versions. Whether you use a manual brush or an electric, make sure you always change your brush or brush head every three months, or sooner if you just had a cold so you don't reinfect yourself.

Flossing – It is very important to floss your teeth at least once per day, (preferably before you go to sleep), to remove food debris and plaque from in between your teeth where your toothbrush cannot reach. Plaque causes tooth decay and can lead to gum disease. Another great reason to floss is that recent studies have shown that flossing helps to prevent a heart attack or stroke. When flossing, be sure to take out a piece of floss about 18 inches long, and gently wrap it around your middle fingers so you have full control and dexterity holding the floss between your thumb and index finger. Then, starting at the base of the gums, work the floss in a circular motion scraping the plaque upwards, away from the gums. Do not forget to wrap the floss around the corner line angles of the tooth where the plaque builds up.

Toothpastes - Toothpastes coupled with the proper brushing action is an effective way to remove plaque, a sticky, harmful film of bacteria that grows on your teeth that causes cavities, gum disease, and eventual tooth loss if not controlled. Toothpastes also contain fluoride, which makes the entire tooth structure more resistant to tooth decay. Toothpastes also help to remove superficial stains and help to leave your mouth with a clean, fresh feeling. It doesn't matter what kind of toothpaste you use, as long as it contains fluoride.

Other Dental Aids- Other dental aids that work very well are pre-brushing rinses, such as Plax, and post brushing antiseptic mouthwashes designed to help kill germs between your teeth. Water Jet Irrigators, such as Waterpiks, are effective for cleaning in between teeth, especially when one does not have the dexterity for flossing properly. Proxybrushes (brushes designed to remove plaque and debris in open areas between the teeth) and Stimudents (very thin wooden toothpick made of orangewood) are also great adjuncts to removing debris that gets trapped between the teeth.

Tongue Scraping - Your tongue is the most retentive surface in your mouth, and is quite adept at harboring bacteria within its Velcro-like surface. It is the anaerobic bacteria and volatile sulfur compounds trapped in these surfaces that give off the oral malodor. Tooth brushing alone does not clean our mouths, and mouth rinses only mask the bad breath for a short period of time. It has been found that 90% of halitosis (bad breath) originates from the mouth, with 80% coming from the posterior third of the tongue. Brushing the posterior of the tongue will stimulate a gag reflex. The only definite way to remove those volatile sulfur compounds is to scrape the tongue with a tongue scraper designed to reach that area.

Question: Should I floss before or after brushing my teeth?

Answer: It is recommended that you floss *after* you brush. Flossing before brushing can be very messy for most people. Additionally, flossing in a mouth that has a lot of debris can only serve to introduce more bacteria into the gum pockets. If one brushes very well, they should be able to better visualize what they are trying to accomplish with the floss.

Question: Can I use baking soda to brush my teeth instead of toothpaste? It seems to work well, but there isn't any fluoride in there.

Answer: Baking Soda, sodium bicarbonate, is one of the least abrasive and most effective tooth cleaners on the market today. Data from various clinical and lab studies show that a toothpaste containing baking soda neutralizes acids and odors, removes plaque and deep tooth stain more readily than other leading toothpastes, and leaves your mouth fresh and feeling very clean. Baking soda is a soft mineral that is very soluble in water, and therefore not very abrasive. In fact, it is less abrasive then most other toothpaste-cleaning agents that are sold.

One can use baking soda to brush their teeth without buying the toothpaste that contains baking soda. It would be more cost effective to do so, however, the toothpaste version would be easier to use (no time wasted dissolving and mixing the powder in water), and it would, most likely, taste better. If you were to use the baking soda version, since it does not contain fluoride, it would be advisable to use an after brushing fluoride rinse to help prevent cavities.

Myth vs. Fact

Myth: My parents had bad teeth, so my dental problems have to be hereditary.

Fact: It is possible your problems may hereditary, but not very likely. Just because your parents had bad teeth doesn't mean that you are doomed to the same fate. In fact, many times a person's dental issues can be traced back to poor home care habits that were taught by those parents who had bad teeth from their poor home care. The bad oral hygiene techniques were passed down, not the bad teeth gene. Only a small percent of patients actually inherited their problems.

20

MISCELLANEOUS

{Sub-categories: Bad Breath (Halitosis), Canker Sores, Cracked Teeth, Dry Mouth (Xerostomia), Oral Piercings, Sleep Apnea, Teeth Grinding and Clenching (Bruxism), Tooth Sensitivity, Glossitis and Geographic Tongue}

Dental Fact...

Diet sodas are just as damaging as regular sodas at weakening tooth enamel.

Important Dental Topics in a category of their own

"Not one for labels"

This chapter explores some very important topics in dentistry. Each of these topics doesn't really fit into any one specific category in dentistry, so they are represented here in this miscellaneous section.

Miscellaneous Oral Problems and Treatments

Bad Breath (Halitosis)

Question: What can I do to prevent bad breath? Do mints, gums, breath sprays and mouth rinses work?

Answer: Be assured that you are not the only one who struggles with this condition. It has been said that bad breath is so common that it is difficult to decide which is normal: individuals who have bad breath or those who do not have it. Bad breath, also referred to as oral malodor or halitosis, is so common a problem that it is estimated that well over a billion dollars are spent on products to combat this widespread condition. Of the 50% of the adult population affected, 90% of the odors were found to be of oral causes and therefore become the responsibility of the dentist to diagnose and treat these individuals.

Many products found in commercial markets simply try to control oral malodor by masking it with minty and fruity scents. Mint candies, gums and most mouthwashes are not powerful enough on their own to combat the foul smelling volatile sulfur compounds, the molecules primarily responsible for oral malodor. At this moment I'm sure that many of you are breathing into your hand to see if you may be one of those affected individuals. Don't bother. One problem associated with bad breath is the inability to self-diagnose. A person with a normal sense of smell usually becomes desensitized to its own stimulants. The majority of individuals with halitosis are often unaware they even have bad breath unless someone around them happens to mention it.

So what can be done? The most effective way to manage oral malodor is by maintaining proper oral hygiene, regular dental cleanings, and diligent brushing of the tongue. Remember, your tongue is the most retentive surface in your mouth, and is quite adept at harboring bacteria within its Velcro-like surface.

Other oral factors that can cause bad breath include food impacted between teeth, faulty restorations, throat infections, food and bacteria caught within the crypts of your tonsils, and unclean dentures. Some non-oral causes may include: post nasal drip, diabetes mellitus, kidney failure, infections of the upper respiratory tract, and, of course, foods such as garlic and onions, which are rich sources of volatile sulfur compounds. Reduced salivation, or dry mouth, has been shown to make one's halitosis more readily perceived.

Dry mouth resulting from mouth breathing or as a side effect of many medications can also be a common cause of bad breath. Sugar-free sour candies may help to stimulate the flow of your saliva, and walking around with a water bottle will help keep your mouth moist. Remember, mints and mouth rinses will mask odor only for a brief duration. Smartmouth is a very effective and promising rinse, with a zinc ion solution that helps to eliminate bad breath for up to 12 hours. If you want to eliminate bad breath, consult with your dentist.

Canker Sores

Question: What are canker sores?

Answer: Canker sores are painful open sores in the mouth (usually less that 1cm) that look like whitish-yellow areas surrounded by a bright red area. They tend to occur more frequently in women than men, and can occur at any age, but typically between the ages of 10 - 40. They can manifest as a single bump or a group of bumps. These sores usually appear on the surface of the gums, roof of the mouth, cheeks, lips and tongue. These sores are completely benign. Symptoms start with a tingling or burning sensation, and progresses to a more painful bump or red spot that eventually becomes an open ulcer. It is possible to develop fever, swollen lymph glands and a general discomfort or malaise, but not for the most part. Within 1-2 weeks the pain will disappear, although canker sores frequently return again.

Question: What causes canker sores?

Answer: Canker sores can be linked to problems with the body's immune system, but often times they are brought about by emotional stress, hormonal changes, menstrual periods, food allergies, spicy foods, and dietary deficiencies of iron, B-12 (cobalamin) and folic acid. These sores may occur after an aggressive tooth cleaning, dental work, or biting one's cheek or tongue. Canker sores often occur in conjunction with a viral infection.

Question: What can I do to prevent and treat canker sores?

Answer: Treatment is usually not necessary, as the canker sores usually go away by themselves. While the canker sore is present, you should avoid eating hot or spicy foods, anything acidic or anything rough and crunchy, as they may cause some discomfort. Prescriptions of corticosteroids or special rinses may be given by your dentist to help with your healing and comfort, but you can also find over-the-counter rinses and medicines that can soothe the painful areas. Warm, salt-water rinses, peroxide rinses or Milk of Magnisia can also be used. In fact, the rinse many dentists prescribe is called the Magic Mouth Rinse, which contains equal parts of viscous lidocaine (as the numbing agent), along with Benadryl and Maalox. In order to help prevent their reoccurrence, keep your resistance up by eating healthy, sleeping well and controlling your stress levels.

Cracked Teeth

Question: What can I do to prevent and treat a cracked tooth?

Answer: There are many factors that could cause a tooth to crack without you even realizing it. Clenching, grinding and unnatural chewing motions can place abnormal stresses on a tooth, leading to a crack. Teeth with large fillings, along with teeth that have lost significant amounts of tooth structure due to aging or wear, are more susceptible to cracking. Even subjecting tooth enamel to extreme variations in temperature, such as drinking hot tea and then sipping ice water, can cause teeth to crack. Of course, traumatic accidents and biting into hard objects or foods are obvious causes of tooth distress. How do you know when your tooth has cracked? Well, many times the crack is not detectable on an X-ray, as it may be small and appear as a hairline fracture running vertically along the tooth. The best way to detect a crack is from your symptoms. If you have sensitivity to cold, heat, air, sweet, or to sticky foods, take note where it is coming from. You may be able to help your dentist diagnose the origin of your problem. Cracked teeth usually hurt more upon the release of your bite than from the pressure of biting itself. Do not be alarmed just because your tooth may be sensitive. Not all sensitivity comes from a cracked tooth, and not all cracked teeth are causes for concern. Tiny cracks are often encountered, and usually do not require any dental treatment. Other times, bonding, onlays, veneers and crowns may be necessary to restore a cracked tooth. A tooth, which is found to be severely cracked, may require root canal therapy or even an extraction. Schedule an appointment with your dentist so that together you can diagnose the origin of your discomfort, and determine which treatment modality will best serve your condition.

Dry Mouth (Xerostomia)

Question: What causes dry mouth (xerostomia)?

Answer: There are many factors that contribute to decreased levels of saliva and developing dry mouth. One of the most common causes is derived from prescription and over-the-counter medications (including antidepressants, decongestants, antihistamines, painkillers and diuretics). Other factors that may cause dry mouth are radiation therapy for head and neck cancers, Sjogren's syndrome (an immune system disorder), salivary gland diseases and diabetes. There are also a number of cases of dry mouth that are associated with pregnancy, menopause and emotional stress.

Question: Why is saliva so important?

Answer: Saliva is the mouth's lubricant. It coats all the soft tissue in the mouth, bathes the teeth to help prevent against cavities and infections, and aids in the digestion of food. When someone has a compromised flow of saliva, various health problems can result. With diminished salivary flow, a person will be more susceptible to yeast infections, gum disease, bad breath, burning sensations in the mouth, tooth decay and can have a difficulty in swallowing.

Question: How do I help a dry mouth (xerostomia)?

Answer: For starters, increasing one's consumption of water may alleviate the symptoms of dry mouth. Other times saliva substitutes may be indicated to keep the soft tissues of the mouth lubricated. Avoiding alcohol (including mouth rinses that contain alcohol), caffeine and carbonated drinks will help to prevent the mouth from becoming too dry. Additionally, sugar-free gums and sour candies may help to stimulate salivary flow. If you do suffer from dry mouth, your dentist may recommend fluoride rinses, pastes, or trays to help prevent against developing cavities and gum disease. There are actually several lines of products specifically designed to help treat a mouth that is chronically dry, including Biotene, which has a line of products (including gums, toothpastes and alcohol-free mouth rinses) designed to stimulate your salivary flow. Smartmouth has a Dry Mouth Activated Oral Rinse that helps to lock in moisture and contains zinc ion technology o help eliminate bad breath for 12 hours. Ask your dentist what they recommend.

Oral Piercings

Question: What are the dental complications of having oral piercings?

Answer: For starters, the piercing of oral structures has a higher than normal risk of infection due to the vast amounts of bacteria that thrive in the mouth. Unfortunately, as body piercing becomes more en vogue, and as individuals run out of body parts to pierce, many are now turning to the mouth, lips and tongue as places to adorn their jewelry. Common symptoms following the piercing of intraoral structures include pain, swelling, infection and an increased salivary flow. Other potential complications include the cracking or fracturing of teeth and restorations; the interference with chewing, swallowing or speaking; and the development of nerve sensitivity as a result of the galvanic currents that arise from the metal jewelry contacting the metal fillings in one's mouth. It is important to point out that a large portion of the population of individuals who choose to pierce their lips, checks and tongue will more than likely undergo one or more of the above listed adverse conditions. There have been a number of patients who have required a root canal or tooth extraction due to the damage caused by their oral piercings. And it is not unheard of to encounter serious secondary infections or even airway obstruction from excessive swelling. It is best to think long and hard before subjecting one's self to this form of art and self-expression.

Sleep Apnea

Question: What is sleep apnea?

Answer: Sleep apnea (the cessation of airflow for more than 10 seconds during sleep) is a very serious and potentially life-threatening condition caused by the periodic collapse of the pharyngeal airway during sleep. Collapse can occur due to a decrease in muscle tone of the pharynx, palate and tongue, or from abnormal anatomy around the level of the soft palate, base of the tongue and lower jaw. During apnea, airflow is restricted despite continued efforts to breathe, until the person is awakened with a gasp of air. It is estimated that 4% of middle aged men and 2% of middle aged women have sleep apnea. This condition is also more prevalent among the obese, and among older individuals.

Question: How can your dentist help to treat your sleep apnea?

Answer: Sleep apnea can be treated non-surgically or surgically. The non-surgical methods include: correcting behavioral measures such as weight loss, elimination of alcohol and sedatives at night, avoiding large, late night meals and avoiding sleeping face up. Oral or dental appliances may be useful in mild to moderate cases of sleep apnea and for improving snoring by repositioning the jaw, tongue and palate to create a better flow of air. Side effects may include an increase in salivation and some TMJ discomfort.

Teeth Grinding and Clenching (Bruxism)

Question: What causes teeth grinding and clenching (bruxism) and what are its manifestations?

Answer: The main causes of teeth grinding and clenching (bruxism) are stress, and a poor bite. People often take out their worries, fears and stress subconsciously, while they sleep, causing the muscles and joints associated with the mouth to become strained and over-worked. These muscles can go into spasm, and the joints can become inflamed and result in pain of the TMJ (temporomandibular joint). Teeth clenching and grinding can also result in the loss of enamel, causing teeth to become more sensitive and causing the eventual need for root canal therapy and crowns. When tooth structure is lost, the bite collapses, resulting in the face to develop an older appearance. Grinding can also cause teeth to fracture and can cause mobility of the teeth. When the bite is off, the muscles and joints can become strained, resulting in TMJ problems and jaw pain. When this happens, neck problems and headaches can arise, and one's posture can become affected. Keep in mind that the chewing muscles can exert a lot of force.

Question: What causes teeth to get shorter over time?

Answer: People do not often notice the subtle wearing down of their tooth structure, which over time can amount to a huge change in the appearance of their smile. Just like you may not notice the sole of your shoe wearing down until you see the hole, your bite can collapse in much the same way. Severe wearing down of the teeth's outer layer (enamel) is often the result from grinding or *bruxing* of the teeth. Acidic conditions (such as acid reflux, bulimia, etc.) can also act to weaken the tooth structure accelerating this wear. Severe wear may become evident on the front teeth, the back teeth or on both, depending on the way one grinds. Excessive wear in the back of the mouth translates to even more wear in the front as the bite collapses. When the front teeth are affected, the teeth start to get more translucent at the top edges, and start to chip away. As these front teeth continue to wear down, and the teeth become shorter, the face begins to take on a much older appearance.

Question: Is it normal for a toddler to grind their teeth? What can be done about it?

Answer: It is not uncommon for toddlers to grind their teeth at night. In fact, about 35% of children do grind their teeth according to some studies. There may be a variety of reasons responsible for their teeth grinding, including: teething pain, malocclusion (when teeth are not meeting properly), and just simply their trying to get used to the new sensation of having teeth. The average age when the grinding may start is at 3 years old, and usually ending by the age of 6. This grinding is not very likely to result in any real damage to their teeth, but you should mention it to your child's dentist to prevent any possible problems from arising.

Although the noise can become quite disturbing, you may just have to wait a period of time for your child to grow out of it. Older children may be fitted with a night guard appliance, although they will probably need to go through a few of them as their teeth and jaws continue to grow.

Tooth Sensitivity

Question: What are the causes of tooth sensitivity?

Answer: Sensitivity of the teeth can occur for many reasons. Some of the causes include:

- ❖ Teeth grinding and clenching
- ❖ Exposed root surfaces due to gum recession or tooth brush abrasion
- ❖ Tooth decay
- ❖ Tooth mobility
- ❖ Tooth cracks or fractures
- ❖ Nerve damage
- ❖ Tooth trauma

Question: What can be done to prevent, reduce or treat tooth sensitivity?

Answer: Often times if you solve the cause of a problem you will eliminate the symptoms. Tooth sensitivity caused by grinding and clenching, can often be eliminated by reducing, eliminating or learning to cope with the stresses encountered in one's life. Tooth sensitivity brought about by malocclusion (improper bite) can be reduced in various ways, including: adjusting one's bite, redoing inadequate restorations, correcting asymmetries and poor jaw position with various removable appliances, and sometimes full mouth reconstruction to restore teeth to their proper levels.

Question: How long should one have to live with sensitive teeth?

Answer: Minor amounts of sensitivity can often be controlled with sensitivity toothpastes, fluoride gels or other types of desensitizing agents. However, if the amount of discomfort that you get from this sensitivity is causing you to change your lifestyle or is a constant source of distress, you should address this sensitivity more definitively. First, you should see your dentist to determine the cause of your sensitivity (i.e. exposed root areas, teeth grinding, fracture, cavities, etc.). Second, take note of what causes the sensitivity (i.e. hot, cold, air, sweets, etc.) and its duration (does it linger, or does it go away after the stimulus is removed?). Often times your dentist can put a layer of bonding over an exposed root, make you a night guard for grinding, or repair a cavity or minor tooth fracture. If the sensitivity still persists, a more involved treatment may be indicated.

Glossitis and Geographic Tongue

Question: What is glossitis?

Answer: Glossitis simply means inflammation of the tongue. Glossitis (a.k.a. burning tongue syndrome) is a condition in which the tongue becomes swollen, tender and changes color. Symptoms may include difficulty with chewing, swallowing or speaking. The papillae (finger-like projections on the surface of the tongue) are lost, causing the tongue to appear smooth. The causes of glossitis include:

❖ Bacterial or viral infections
❖ Trauma from burns, rough edges of teeth or dental appliances, etc.
❖ Exposure to certain stimuli such as tobacco, alcohol, hot foods, or spices
❖ Dry mouth associated with disorders such as Sjogren's syndrome
❖ Allergic reaction to toothpaste, mouthwash, breath fresheners, and certain dyes and plastics
❖ Disorders such as iron deficiency anemia, B-vitamin deficiencies, oral lichen planus, aphthous ulcers, syphilis, and others
❖ Yeast infection

Treatment for glossitis includes:

❖ Good oral hygiene
❖ Dietary changes and supplements (especially when treating a glossitis caused by anemia and nutritional deficiencies)
❖ Avoiding irritants (such as hot or spicy foods, alcohol, and tobacco)
❖ Antibiotics, but only if the glossitis is due to an infection.

If symptoms of glossitis persist for longer than 10 days, contact your dental care provider.

Call your health care provider ASAP if tongue swelling is severe or breathing, speaking, chewing, or swallowing is difficult.

Question: What is the difference between glossitis and geographic tongue?

Answer: When the papillae (pinkish-white, finger-like bumps on the surface of the tongue) are lost, it creates a bald and shiny condition of the tongue called glossitis. When this usually benign condition changes in size, location and appearance, it is then termed migratory glossitis or geographic tongue. Geographic tongue is a harmless condition, where patches on the surface of the tongue are missing papillae and appear as smooth, red "islands," often with slightly raised borders. These patches (lesions) give the tongue a map-like, or geographic, appearance. The lesions often heal in one area and then move (migrate) to a different part of your tongue. Although geographic tongue may look alarming, it doesn't cause health problems and isn't associated with infection or cancer. Geographic tongue can sometimes cause tongue discomfort and increased sensitivity to certain substances.

Myth vs. Fact

Myth: Diet sodas are not bad for my teeth.

Fact: Diet soda does not contribute to the development of cavities due to the lack of sugar. However, the acid in diet soda has the potential to contribute to the breakdown of the tooth's enamel. The pH of regular and diet soda ranges from 2.47-3.35. The PH in our mouth is normally about 6.2 to 7.0 slightly more acidic than water. Once the PH reaches below the range of 5.2 to 5.5, the acid begins to dissolve the hard enamel of our teeth. The phosphoric and citric acids within the diet soda contribute to that acidity. Additionally, when a person drinks regular soda, and combines the acid with the sugar, rampant decay will ensue.

21

ALTERNATIVE DENTAL CARE

Fun Fact...

There are 60 herbs commonly cited for treatment of dental problems in ancient Chinese medical books.

Open your mind before opening your mouth

"Alternative therapies today may become conventional therapies tomorrow"

Alternative remedies and treatments, when used appropriately, can be a great adjunct to traditional dental care and help one to utilize their immune system more efficiently. Natural healing has been a valid alternative for centuries, but it is often misunderstood, abused and misused, resulting in its lack of acceptance within certain circles of western science and medicine. Interestingly enough, some of our traditional medicines were derived from these natural substances. We may come to find that some of what is alternative today may become conventional tomorrow. As we start to recognize the popularity of these alternative treatments and begin to try them ourselves, we must remember to tell our healthcare provider what we are taking, as these natural remedies can still have interactions with the medications that we may be prescribed. This chapter seeks to explain what alternative dental care is all about and answer some of the most frequently asked questions on this subject.

Alternative Dental Care

Question: Why Alternative Care?

Answer: As individuals achieve a heightened sense of awareness for improving their overall health, they turn to alternative therapies either instead of, or in addition to, traditional medications and treatments. Natural healing has been a valid form of treatment for centuries. It is the quackery, abuse and misuse of natural substances that may be hindering the development of alternative therapies as an acceptable means of treating diseases. Some of what is alternative today may become conventional tomorrow. After all, is it so inconceivable that nature could have created substances that are capable of achieving the same results that have been developed by modern science? Keep in mind that there are a number of western medicines that have been derived from natural substances. In 2735 BC, a Chinese emperor recommended an extract from the Ma Huang plant (known as ephedra in the western world) as treatment for respiratory illness. Today the chemical ephedrine is extracted from the plant and used as decongestants (pseudoephedrine). Codeine, derived from opium, has long been used as an analgesic and cough suppressant. Other plant-derived drugs include digitalis (a heart strengthener) and Vincristine (an anti-tumor drug).

Studies have found that a third of the people polled admitted to using at least one alternative within the past year. Dental health care providers should have the following questions on their medical/ drug history form: "Are you currently taking any herbal or natural homeopathic remedies?" and "If so, are you under the supervision of an alternative therapist?" If these questions are not one of the questions on the form, then please make sure to tell your dentist (and other doctors) exactly what you are taking.

Question: What are some alternative therapies for gum inflammation?

Answer: It has been proven in studies that when placing gauze soaked in aloe vera gel or liquid over an extraction site or periodontal surgical site, the post-operative pain, swelling and bleeding are significantly reduced. Aloe vera (known by the Egyptians as "The Plant of Immortality") has been used internally and externally since at least 400 BC. It has been confirmed by clinical research that aloe vera: (1) anesthetizes tissue, (2) kills bacteria, (3) kills viruses, (4) kills fungi, (5) helps stop bleeding, (6) is an antipyretic (reduces heat), (7) is an anti-inflammatory, (8) is a capillary dilator, (9) is an enhancer of cell growth, and (10) is a tissue moisturizer. Aloe vera has been shown to treat systemic oral lichen planus, angular chelitis (irritations around the corners of the mouth), dry lips and herpes.

In addition to aloe vera, there are some herbal remedies that can suppress inflammation with fewer side effects than currently available pharmaceuticals. Echinacea has gained popularity in the United States, being hailed by some to be an immune system "booster," an antimicrobial agent and an antiviral agent. Goldenseal has been used for its anti-inflammatory and anti-microbial properties, and immune-strengthening properties. Grapefruit Seed Extract (GSE) is a bioflavonoid complex that possesses anti-inflammatory activities and inhibits the release of certain compounds that influence inflammation. Other anti-inflammatory agents include Calendula, Bloodroot, and Wild yam, Licorice, Fenugreek and Figwort.

Question: Are these alternative remedies safe?

Answer: When taken appropriately, herbal and homeopathic remedies can have a wonderful healing effect on the body. Like many western drugs, herbal remedies have potential risks, side effects, and drug interactions that can interfere with traditional western medicines and affect the safe practice of dentistry. The Food and Drug Administration (FDA) currently regulates prescription and over-the-counter drugs but not herbal preparations. As a result, it is critical that the dental profession continue to increase its level of understanding and education about these alternative medications and treatments so that these new generations of dental patients are treated in a safe and effective manner.

Question: How does one avoid taking antibiotics unnecessarily?

Answer: It has been well stated that the individual who successfully counters infections without antibiotics probably utilizes his/her immune system more appropriately than he/she would otherwise. While antibiotics definitely have their place, they are overused, and overprescribed. In the presence of an acute infection or as a prophylactic measure to prevent against bacterial endocarditis, for those who are susceptible, it is of the utmost importance. We are, however, living in a society where the average doctor prescribes more antibiotics than are necessary; 50% of the time they may not even be required.

22

KEEPING COSTS DOWN

Fun Fact...

Oral disease affects 3.9 billion people worldwide with untreated tooth decay.

The 10 best ways to keep dental costs down

"The best and least expensive form of dentistry is making sure the right thing is done extremely well the first time"

One of the main contributing factors to the avoidance of dental care, aside from fear and anxiety, is the cost of dentistry. Yes, dentistry can be quite costly even with insurance; however, the cost of avoidance is much greater. Especially when you consider that routine dental care can maintain your oral health as well as your body's health. Regular dental examinations can alert you to dental and medical problems that you may not realize are starting to occur. In the end, there is no greater investment than in yourself and your health.

Keeping Costs Down

Question: What are the 10 best ways to keep dental costs down?

Answer: One of the main reasons for people avoiding dental care, (aside from their fears, anxiety and lack of time), is the expense. Dentistry can be expensive for many people, but there are ways to minimize these costs and still get the treatment you need and want. The following are 10 ways you can keep your dental costs down:

❖ **Catch it early!** - A small pinpoint cavity that can be cleaned out without any anesthesia and filled very conservatively and inexpensively will save a lot of money in the long run. When left untreated, that tiny cavity can become a large cavity that requires a more expensive restoration such as a multiple surface filling, an inlay/onlay (restorations usually made by a dental lab that fill in missing areas of tooth structure when an area is too large for a filling) or a crown. Additionally, if ignored further, that area of decay can extend into the nerve creating the need for root canal therapy. If the decay extends beneath the gums, closer to the level of bone, a crown lengthening may be necessary to lower the gums and bone to allow the crown to grab onto some good tooth structure. This procedure is a minor surgical procedure performed by a periodontist. Sometimes the decay can extend far beneath the gums and bone, resulting in the need for an extraction and subsequent bridge or implant. All these treatments add up, which is why it is better to practice preventative dentistry and have biomimetic restorations instead of more invasive and expensive procedures.

❖ **Have regular cleanings** - Routine cleanings can save you many thousands in periodontal (gum) work, implants and bridges later on. During a regular dental checkup your dentist or hygienist will examine your gums for any inflammation and measure the "pockets" between the gums and teeth. Normal, healthy gums will have pockets of 3 millimeters or less, but as plaque starts to accumulate, the gums get more inflamed and start to pull away from the teeth causing deeper pockets to form. As deeper pockets form, more plaque accumulates, (which hardens into tartar over a short period of time), and the gums recede more in response to the tartar. The downward spiral continues, and eventually the bone surrounding the teeth starts to recede along with the gums. As this process continues, teeth become increasingly more mobile, and eventually they can be lost. The cost of gum surgeries, implants, bridges, etc., can really add up. Your regular dental visits and cleanings are your best insurance policy.

❖ **Biomimetic Dentistry and Preventative Care** – Often times the best way to save money is to be conservative, proactive and preventative. Biomimetic dentistry can save you both money, time and tooth structure, often times avoiding invasive and expensive procedures such as root canals, crowns, extractions and implants. Know your options, do your research and find a Biomimetic dentist near you who understands the importance of saving all good tooth structure. Take digital X-rays and catch things when they are small and less involved. Have regular dental check-ups and seal up any areas that may be more prone to developing cavities.

❖ **Inexpensive Smile Makeovers** – So you've always wanted that perfect, white smile, or at least an improved version of your own, but can't afford to spend $10,000 or up (usually way up) for porcelain veneers. There are other options, including enamel reshaping, bonding and whitening. **Enamel reshaping** is the reshaping and contouring of the enamel of the teeth to remove sharp edges and uneven characteristics of the teeth, and to give the illusion that the teeth are straighter than they really are. This reshaping of the tooth's enamel lends to an improvement of the overall appearance of a smile, correcting the flaws that catch one's eye, such as a tooth that is longer than the others, or an obvious overlapping or rotation of the teeth due to crowding. Enamel reshaping is a conservative process, often combined with some bonding, does not require any anesthesia, and is relatively quick and painless. **Bonding** uses composite resin to restore chipped or broken teeth, fill in gaps, fix cavities and reshape or recolor your smile. The same material used for bonding is used for making tooth-colored fillings, which appear more natural. Your dentist applies the resin and sculpts, colors and shapes it to provide a pleasing result. A special light, operating at a specific wavelength, hardens the material, which is then adjusted and polished. Bonding differs from veneers in that bonding can be done within a single visit, while veneers require a dental lab to manufacture the restoration. Additionally, bonded restorations are much less expensive than veneering, since there are no lab costs involved. Bonded restorations are usually very conservative when it comes to reducing tooth structure, and can also be used to protect overexposed root surfaces in order to reduce tooth sensitivity. **Teeth Whitening** is a way to reverse the signs of age in teeth, and remove the years of cumulative stain from coffee, wine, soda, teriyaki sauce, tomato sauce, etc. These unsightly stains can be removed quickly, safely, and with minimal discomfort utilizing in-office whitening systems, custom home trays, and over-the-counter products. When enamel reshaping, bonding and whitening are combined, they can create a very effective smile makeover without having to spend a fortune.

❖ **Be a Teaching Case** – Certain cosmetic dentists may be interested in performing your smile makeover in front of other doctors and dental students as a teaching case or so that they may document the procedure for an article they wish to publish. Many times the dentist will only charge you the lab costs, which can save you many thousands of dollars. Sometimes the dentist may offer to assume all costs for this, especially when the dental lab they use also wishes to use your photos for marketing their service.

❖ **When a tooth is lost, maintain that space** - Many people prioritize their dental health by taking care of the teeth they can see when they smile and put off care for the teeth they do not see. A number of patients will choose to spend their money whitening their front teeth, instead of putting those funds towards restoring a compromised back tooth. When that back tooth fails, and needs to be removed, the space often gets left there without a bridge or an implant to help fill in the space. Empty spaces in the back are a big deal! When you have an empty space, the adjacent teeth can drift and tilt, causing spacing, gum pockets, and loss of bone. Opposing teeth will tend to slowly erupt out of its socket in attempt to meet up with another tooth. Additionally, if multiple teeth are lost in the back of the mouth, it causes an additional stress on the other teeth, resulting in the enamel to wear faster. In the case of heavy grinders, missing teeth in the back can cause front teeth to wear, chip and break, causing their bite to collapse, and contribute to an unattractive smile. It is recommended to invest in that implant or that bridge to maintain the space, even if you need to finance the costs. The space can also be maintained temporarily with a removable appliance if the cost of an implant or bridge is too prohibitive. Either way, maintaining that space will save you many thousands later on.

❖ **<u>Choose the right dentist the first time</u>** – Many people choose a dentist just because their location is convenient, or because they are the least expensive. This is not the way to go about selecting a dentist. These factors may play a role in your final decision; however, if you choose right the first time you will save money and time in the long run. Conversely, a dentist who charges a large fee does not necessarily provide greater dental care. Also, you should avoid choosing a dentist based on flashy advertisements, paid for media placements, or misleading claims that promise certain results within a certain time frame. Instead, you should ask for a referral from someone you know and trust. Once you have a name, you should Google them, check their background, affiliations, dental society standings, etc. Take the time to review their before and after photos, patient testimonials and learn about their practice (is it clean, up to date, and practicing proper infection control techniques?). The dentist you choose should be committed to a high standard of ethics, and you should feel that your health and care means more to them than your wallet. Ideally the dentist you choose should understand and practice tooth conserving Biomimetic dentistry, as avoiding and preventing invasive dental procedures can help to save your money and your teeth in the long run.

* **Prevention is Key** – Sealants, Fluorides and X-rays are some of the preventative measures that will save a lot of money for you and your family down the road. **Sealants** have become one of the biggest breakthroughs in terms of dental prevention. They are used to protect teeth from decay and are appropriate as soon as a posterior tooth erupts. The chewing surfaces of these back teeth have many pits and grooves that can trap food debris and cause cavities. **Fluoride** helps to prevent against tooth decay by strengthening the tooth's enamel and making it more resistant to acids and harmful bacteria. With fluoride, your teeth become more resistant to developing tooth decay, which can lead to fairly expensive restorations when left untreated. **X-rays** provide valuable information that your dentist could not detect otherwise. With the help of X-rays, your dentist can look at what is happening in areas that are not visible clinically. X-rays can detect cavities between the teeth, and can depict approximately how deep a cavity extends relative to the nerve. They can also help diagnose periodontal disease, abscesses, cysts, tumors, developmental abnormalities and infections in the bone. Avoiding X-rays because of their cost would be a mistake, since the little problems that they can detect will become bigger ones when left undetected.

* **Wear a night guard** - Whether you have all natural teeth, or have just spent a small fortune restoring or cosmetically enhancing your smile, a night guard may be the best

way to look after your investment. A night guard can prevent the porcelain from your crowns and veneers from breaking, and prevent their wear if you grind your teeth. A night guard is a device most often recommended as the first line of treatment for teeth grinding and TMJ pain. It is usually worn while you sleep to prevent damaging your teeth by the clenching or grinding associated with either the psychological aspects of stress, one's abnormal bite, a sleep disorder, or a combination of the above. Grinding can wear away the surfaces of your teeth causing them to become painful or loose. Once the enamel is lost, it could become quire costly and frustrating to have to undergo root canal therapy and the fabrication of crowns. You won't want to look back years from now regretting how you wound up spending thousands of dollars and time on dental work that could have been prevented with a few hundred dollar night guard. Remember, we only get one set of adult teeth, so please protect your smile.

❖ **Financing your dentistry** – There are many types of payment plan options available to enable you to undergo the dental care that you have been putting off. Most of these plans (such as Care Credit, Dental Fee Plan or Chase bank) have rates that are lower than what you would pay with your credit card, and many have interest free financing available for up to 2 years. For example, let's say you are interested in getting *Invisalign®* to straighten your teeth, but can't afford the $4,800 it would cost, you could get financing through Chase that would allow you to pay $200 per month interest free for 2 years. Ask your dentist if they participate in any of these payment plan options.

23

CHOOSING A DENTIST

Dental Fact...

The number one reason for switching
dentists is due to a lack of trust.

Take the time, Do your research

*"Trust takes years to build...
and seconds to break"*

Choosing the right dentist is a very important decision to make,
and not one that should be determined just because it is cheaper or
more convenient. The right dentist will spend the time to educate
you and make you feel comfortable with your dental care both in
and out of their office. Choosing a reputable dentist will also wind
up saving you time and money in the long run. So how do you
choose the right dentist and what qualities should you look for? This
chapter will answer those questions and more to guide you towards
making the best decision for your dental health care needs.

Choosing a Dentist

Question: How does one go about choosing a dentist?

Answer: Many people choose a dentist just because their location
is convenient, or because they are the least expensive. This is not

the way to go about selecting a dentist. These factors may play a role in your final decision; however, if you choose right the first time you will save money and time in the long run. Conversely, a dentist who charges a large fee does not necessarily provide greater dental care. Also, you should avoid choosing a dentist based on flashy advertisements, paid for media placements, or misleading claims that promise certain results within a certain time frame. Instead, you should ask for a referral from someone you know and trust. Once you have a name, you should Google them, check their background, affiliations, dental society standings, etc. Take the time to review their before and after photos, patient testimonials and learn about their practice (is it clean, up to date, and practicing proper infection control techniques?). The dentist you choose should be committed to a high standard of ethics, and you should feel that your health and care means more to them than your wallet.

Question: Which qualities should I look for in a dentist?

Answer: You should look for a dentist who has the ability to put you at ease, and who takes the time to listen to your concerns and answer your questions. Your dentist should take pride in what they do, and recognize the importance of educating their patients. Ideally he or she should practice tooth conserving Biomimetic dentistry and preventative dental care. He or she should be up to date with their continuing education and technology, wear loupes (special glasses with magnification and built-in light source) to enable better vision, maintain a clean work environment, and treat their staff well. You should always feel that YOU are the first priority, not your wallet.

Question: How do I find a dentist while traveling?

Answer: If you should require dental services while traveling, the first place to call would be your dental office to see if they can help locate a reputable dental provider in the area where you are traveling. If you are not able to secure a recommendation that way, you may contact the local dental society, dental school or hospital, or ask for a referral from a dependable source, and then research them online if possible. You may also visit www.aobmd.org to search for a *Certified* Biomimetic dentist near you.

Question: When should I see a general dentist versus seeing a specialist?

Answer: No dentist is great at everything. While a dental degree allows one to practice any aspect of dentistry, the best dentists are those who are willing to refer you to someone else when the work required is beyond their scope of expertise. For example, unless a general dentist is specially trained, and habitually removes impacted wisdom teeth, you are better off seeing an oral surgeon. If you are interested in having braces, inquire about the dentist's experience with that particular procedure, because more times than not, an orthodontist (while usually more expensive), will be better suited to give you the desired results without the complications.

Question: What's the difference between a DDS and a DMD?

Answer: There is no difference between the DDS (Doctor of Dental Surgery) and DMD (Doctor of Dental Medicine) degrees. The difference is only a matter of semantics. Most dental schools award the DDS degree; however, there are some that award a DMD degree. The level of education and degrees given are valued the same.

About the author: Dr. Marc Lazare

Dr. Lazare's - The Patient's Guide to Biomimetic Dentistry and Smile Design - is written by Dr. Marc Lazare, an internationally renowned lecturer, dental columnist, featured author in peer reviewed dental journals, teacher, consultant, inventor, and President of Cosmetic Innovations, Inc. Dr. Lazare is well regarded by his peers, recognized as an authority on Biomimetic and Cosmetic Dentistry and also known by many as 'Dentist to the Stars.'

Dr. Lazare has been a member of the clinical faculty at the **NYU College of Dentistry** and has been on the teaching staff at **North Shore University Hospital** since 1998. He had previously graduated as Chief Resident at North Shore University Hospital, having spent 2 years of residency there. Dr. Lazare started the Teeth Whitening Division at North Shore University Hospital utilizing the latest technologies. Dr. Lazare is President and Founder of **Cosmetic Innovations, Inc.**, a company selling such dental products as *Veneer Styx* (a device for positioning porcelain laminate veneers) and *Inlay/Onlay Styx* (a device for trying-in and seating inlays, onlays and posterior ceramic crowns), both of which he invented.

Veneer Styx, rated "Top 100 New Products of 2005" – *Dentistry Today* and "Top Technique for 2004" - *Dental Products Report.* His *Inlay/Onlay Styx*, was written up in *Dental Products Report* as one of the "Top New Products of 2005" and was featured as one of the "Top 100 Distinctive Products of 2006" - *Dental Products Report*

Dr. Lazare was the elected **President** of the **Academy of Biomimetic Dentistry** and has also served on its Executive Board for many years. He is also the **Founder** and **President** of the **Lazare Institute for Biomimetics and Smile Design**.

Dr. Lazare is also the developer of the **Dental Expert**, **Pediatric Dental Expert** and **Dental Clinic** Apps for the iPhone, iTouch and iPad. The **Dental Expert** app is a patient's guide to understanding all aspects of dentistry and its procedures. Additionally, he has been a columnist for 5 different magazines, has been published in numerous other magazines and dental journals, and lectures extensively on Biomimetic Dentistry, Smile Design, teeth whitening, porcelain veneers and other esthetic techniques, along with speaking about the importance of nutrition as it applies to dentistry. Dr. Lazare holds a B.A. from the **University of Pennsylvania**, and a D.D.S. degree from **New York University College of Dentistry**. Dr. Lazare earned the designation "**Master**" of the **Academy of General Dentistry** (MAGD), a title earned by less than 1% of the dentists in the United States. He also is a **Fellow** in the **Academy of General Dentistry**, the **Academy of Biomimetic Dentistry** and the **International Academy for Dental-Facial Esthetics**. Dr. Lazare maintains a dental practice in New York City.

To see the complete Curriculum Vitae for Dr. Marc Lazare, feel free to visit his website at: www.drmarclazare.com

Dentistry is an art and science that is always changing and advancing.

Disclaimer

The information provided in this book is not a substitute for professional dental advice, diagnosis or treatment; it is intended for informational purposes only. This book is meant to educate the public so that they can have an informative conversation with their dentist, and to help people understand the various treatment options available in dentistry today.

Copyright Protection Notice:

Contact Us:

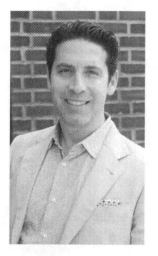

Marc Lazare, D.D.S.
115 East 61st Street
Suite 14A
New York, NY 10065

Office: 212.861.2599
e-mail: office@drmarclazare.com
Website: www.drmarclazare.com

 http://www.twitter.com/marclazaredds

 http://www.facebook.com/marclazaredds

 http://www.instagram.com/drmarclazare

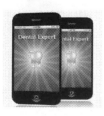 **Dental Expert** App developed by Dr. Lazare for your iPhone, iTouch or iPad